MULTIPLE SCLEROSIS

Questions and Answers for Patients and Loved Ones

Jonathan Howard, MD

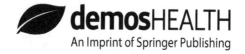

demosHEALTH

An Imprint of Springer Publishing

Visit our website at www.springerpub.com

ISBN: 9780826177469
ebook ISBN: 9780826177476

Acquisitions Editor: Beth Barry
Compositor: diacriTech, Chennai

© 2019 Demos Health.
Demos Health is an imprint of Springer Publishing Company, LLC.

Medical information provided by Demos Health, in the absence of a visit with a health care professional, must be considered as an educational service only. This book is not designed to replace a physician's independent judgment about the appropriateness or risks of a procedure or therapy for a given patient. Our purpose is to provide you with information that will help you make your own health care decisions.

The information and opinions provided here are believed to be accurate and sound, based on the best judgment available to the authors, editors, and publisher, but readers who fail to consult appropriate health authorities assume the risk of injuries. The publisher is not responsible for errors or omissions. The editors and publisher welcome any reader to report to the publisher any discrepancies or inaccuracies noticed.

Contact us to receive discount rates on bulk purchases.
We can also customize our books to meet your needs.
For more information please contact: sales@springerpub.com

Printed in the United States of America.
18 19 20 21 22 / 5 4 3 2 1

CONTENTS

PREFACE

This guide is intended for patients with MS and their loved ones. I hope that it will help patients learn more about their disease and what they can do to lead unencumbered lives. The field of MS changes rapidly. In less than a decade, six new medications for MS have been approved by the FDA. Every few months there is a new discovery that renders a part of this guide out of date. This is good news. I hope one day soon a cure will make this guide useful only to medical historians.

For further information on a wide variety of topics, please use the resources found at the National Center for Biotechnology Information (U.S. National Library of Medicine/PubMed Health) and National Multiple Sclerosis Society websites.

ACKNOWLEDGMENTS

First and foremost, I would like to thank my patients. They are my teachers. Their strength and resiliency will never cease to amaze me. I would also like to honor the memory of Joseph Herbert, who established the NYU MS Center and gave me my first real job.

I would also like to thank several people for their valuable contributions to this guide: Lana Zhovtis Ryerson, Lauren Krupp, Lisa Laing, Benoit Peyronnet, Benjamin Brucker, Kimberly Sackheim, Leigh Charvet, Heather Menzer, Estelle Gallo, Dori Goldman, and Elaine Toskos.

I would like to thank Beth Barry and her team at Springer Publishing for their vision and support.

As always, I want to thank my loving wife Robin for making this all possible. Thanks as well to Nellie for always being there.

1 AN INTRODUCTION TO MS

1. What Are the Worst Symptoms for Newly Diagnosed Patients?

There is no question in my mind that the worst symptoms for almost all newly diagnosed patients are anxiety and fear. Most MS patients are young, healthy people at the time they are diagnosed. Many have not seen a doctor for many years when the symptoms of MS begin to hit them out of nowhere. Naturally, questions arise about the future: Will I be able to continue to walk, to work, to have a family? For many newly diagnosed patients, the anxiety far outweighs whatever symptoms they may have experienced that lead to the diagnosis. In thinking about this, I am reminded of a patient of mine who suffered a spinal cord injury many years ago. He will never walk again, but from a psychiatric standpoint, he long ago adjusted to his illness and is doing well. Many of my patients will never suffer this level of disability. However, they are faced with uncertainty and live in fear of an unpredictable disease.

Although MS is obviously a significant disease for many people, I hope that with newer and more powerful treatments we are able to continually prevent disability and relieve the symptoms many patients feel. I do not want patients to think that they are made of glass or that they are a different species. As much as possible, I want them to try to lead the same life they led the day before they were diagnosed.

2. What Is MS?

MS is a disorder of the central nervous system, which is composed of the brain and spinal cord. It affects about 1 in 750 people in the United States, which means there are approximately 400,000 Americans currently living with the illness. Around the world, there are about 2.5 million people with the disease. More recent research suggests that these numbers are a vast underestimate, and that nearly 1 million people have MS in the United States alone.

MS typically affects people between the ages of 15 and 40, though occasionally people are diagnosed outside of this age range. Aside from trauma, it is the major cause of neurological disability in young people. Once MS has been diagnosed, it is not possible to provide anything other than a very general prognosis, though there are certain risk factors associated with an aggressive disease course. It is a mysterious illness. No one knows what causes it, though certain risk factors have been identified.

3. *Neuroscience Basics*

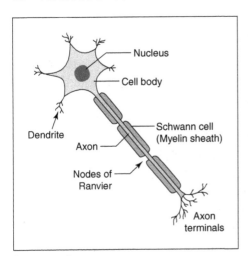

Anatomy of a neuron.

To get a general understanding of what happens in MS, it is important to review some basic neuroscience. Neurons, the main cells in the brain, are composed of a cell body, called the soma, and a tail, called the axon. Axons are the means by which neurons communicate with each other and their structure can be compared to a telephone cord. The axon is the wire at the center of the cord. Each axon has a protective coating composed of fats and lipids, termed the myelin sheath. Myelin is made by cells called oligodendrocytes. Myelin allows electricity to conduct much faster along axons, permitting rapid communication between cells. More specifically, myelin allows an electrical signal to "jump" along an axon (at spaces called nodes of Ranvier), in a process called saltatory conduction.

The soma, or cell body, of neurons of neurons are in the outer part of the brain, called the cortex or grey matter, while the axons and myelin are in the inner part of

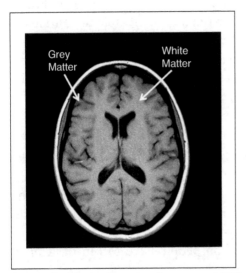

Grey and white matter seen in a normal MRI.

the brain, called the white matter.

4. What Happens in MS?

MS is considered an immune-mediated disorder, meaning that the immune system attacks healthy parts of the body. In MS, the primary target is the myelin sheath, though with advanced disease the axons can also be damaged. When this happens, conduction within the nervous system slows down or stops entirely, and patients develop neurological symptoms. Unlike many autoimmune diseases, no pathological antibody has ever been discovered. There are also no blood tests to diagnose MS. Although MS has traditionally been considered a disease of the white matter, abnormalities of the grey matter have become recognized as playing an important role as well. MS only affects the central nervous system; the peripheral nerves in the arms and legs are completely spared.

5. What Causes MS?

One of the most common questions is what causes MS. The short answer is that no one knows for sure, and there is no single cause. It's like asking why someone is rich; unless that person won the lottery, there is likely no single answer. There are some known risk factors, however.

GENETICS: Genes play a role in MS, though they are not the determining factor as to whether a person will develop the disease or not. Most people are the first in their families to have the disease. If a first-degree relative, such as a sibling or a parent, has MS, the odds that a person will have the illness are about 3% to 5%. If both parents have the disease, there is about a 12% chance that their child will have it. Even in identical twins who share the same DNA, the odds of one twin developing MS if the other has it are only 34% for women and 5% for men. For fraternal (non-identical twins) the risk is only about 5%.

A common fear among people with MS is that it could be passed on to their children. In the United States, the overall risk of developing MS is about 1 in 750 people. So, while the rate of MS for people with affected family members is substantially higher than that of the general population, the vast majority of people with MS have children who do not develop the disease.

The most common genes linked to MS are involved in the human leukocyte antigen system, which plays a role in the immune system. Presently, over 200 genetic loci have been linked to MS. Most of these genes were discovered in the last 4 years.

The advances in the genetics of MS has recently expanded significantly and will serve to further our understanding of the disease. There are many diseases, both neurological and otherwise, where the genetics are almost entirely understood but there is no cure.

For MS and many other immune-mediated diseases, the finding of over 200 genes linked to the illness makes understanding and putting these discoveries to practical use much more difficult. Clearly genes play a role in MS, but they are not the major determinant in disease development. As stated previously, if one identical twin has the illness, the chances that the twin will have the illness are less than 50%. Since identical twins share the exact same DNA, some unknown factor must influence who develops MS and who does not. Moreover, these genes do not provide a prognosis about the severity level of MS.

I suspect that, in the future, genetic testing will play a powerful role in determining who is at risk for developing MS and which treatments will be best for that person. Unfortunately, the science just isn't there today.

SEX: As with most autoimmune illnesses, MS is more than twice as common in women than in men. A report from Canada shows that this imbalance has become even more pronounced in recent years for unclear reasons.

RACE: MS has traditionally been thought to not occur equally in all ethnic groups. Caucasians tend to have the highest rate of the illness, while other races have a lower rate. However, recent research suggests that there is not a large difference among races in incidence of MS, at least in the United States. In black people from Africa, the disease is rare, though not unheard of.

ENVIRONMENTAL FACTORS: The risk of getting MS depends on where a person spends the first 15 years of life. People who live near the Equator have very low rates of MS, but the rate increases the farther one travels away from the Equator. The rate of MS in Ohio is almost double the rate in Texas. There are several theories as to why this might be, but the most popular one is that people who live near the Equator have higher rates of exposure to ultraviolent light, which the body requires to make vitamin D. Low vitamin D levels have been linked to MS. For example, in one study of 800,000 women from Finland, the women with the lowest vitamin D levels had double the MS risk, while those with the highest levels had the lowest risk. Another study found that women exposed to more sunlight during childhood had a lower risk of MS. Currently, vitamin D is being explored as a possible preventive treatment in those people with a strong family history of MS.

EXPOSURE TO INFECTIOUS AGENTS: Infectious agents have long been suspected to be a cause of MS, though no pathogen has been definitively shown to cause the disease. Certain "outbreaks" of MS have occurred, most notably in the Faroe Islands, a small group of islands in the North Atlantic Ocean. Multiple cases of MS occurred there after British soldiers occupied the islands during World War II.

The strongest evidence that an infection predisposes people to MS exists for the Epstein-Barr virus (EBV), which causes mononucleosis. Although the majority of the population has evidence of exposure to EBV, the rate is almost 100% in patients with MS. Exposure to the varicella zoster virus, which causes chickenpox and shingles, has also been implicated in causing MS. More recently, in 2013, researchers identified a bacterium, *Clostridium perfringens* type B, which seems to be related to MS.

Other research indicates that certain infections may help prevent MS, a theory known as the hygiene hypothesis. While it is wonderful that children no longer die of infectious diseases at high rates (at least in wealthy countries), growing up in a relatively sterile environment may lead to more autoimmune diseases. Indeed, one of the more adventurous treatments for MS and other autoimmune disorders is infecting people with parasitic worms in the hope that this will help dampen down the immune response.

OBESITY: In 2013, a study found that obese girls are at greater risk of developing MS. According to the study, the risk was more than one and one-half times higher for overweight girls, almost two times higher in moderately obese girls, and almost four times higher in extremely obese girls. Several other studies have found similar findings. This is likely related to hormonal changes that occur as a result of obesity. The finding that obesity is linked to MS is not as strong in boys.

SODIUM INTAKE: In 2013, a study found that a high sodium diet was linked to the onset of MS. However, another study in 2017 found that there was no such risk.

CONCUSSION: One study from 2017 found that concussions in adolescence, particularly repeated concussions, were associated with an increased risk of MS

SMOKING: The main behavioral factor that leads to MS is that old demon— cigarette smoking—which nearly doubles the risk of developing MS.

In summary, there is no single cause of MS. Rather, it is an illness that occurs in genetically vulnerable individuals exposed to certain environmental conditions. Patients should know that they did not cause their MS. Many MS patients led the healthiest lifestyles imaginable prior to their diagnosis—some professional athletes and dancers have been diagnosed. In contrast, people who smoke, use drugs, eat only junk food, and never exercise are certainly not leading healthy lifestyles. They have much higher rates of cancer and cardiovascular disease, but they do not necessarily have a higher risk of MS. Put another way, if I were an evil doctor who set out to purposefully give someone MS, I would fail. More work remains to be done to illuminate the causes of MS and more discoveries are on the horizon.

Finally, it is important to know what does *not* cause MS. There is no compelling evidence that stress, "toxins," or an unhealthy diet can cause MS. Vaccinations have also been definitively ruled out as a cause of MS.

6. How Is MS Diagnosed?

In medical school, every doctor is taught that the key to a correct diagnosis is obtaining a comprehensive history and performing a thorough physical examination, with radiographic and laboratory tests serving as invaluable aids. The diagnosis of MS is no different. The key to diagnosing MS is to identify two separate episodes of neurological dysfunction that have lasted at least 24 hours and occurred at different points in time (at least 30 days apart) in different parts of the central nervous system. This is technically referred to as dissemination in space and dissemination in time.

In patients who provide a history of two separate neurological relapses with evidence on physical exam of two or more lesions, no further evidence is required to diagnosis MS. However, many patients will come to the neurologist after having had a single episode of neurological dysfunction. Once a patient presents with a neurological symptom suggestive of MS, most neurologists will order a magnetic resonance image (MRI) of the brain and spinal cord. If this reveals lesions typical of MS, further tests are usually unnecessary. However, if the MRI is not typical for MS, a lumbar puncture might be necessary to look for a marker of inflammation known as oligoclonal bands (discussed in the following) in the central nervous system. Only if certain abnormalities are present on these tests can the diagnosis of MS be made. For example, if an MRI shows evidence of both old and new lesions (MRIs are discussed more in the following), this satisfies the criteria for separation in space and time, and a diagnosis of MS can be made in a patient who has had a single clinical event. If such lesions are not present, then patients with only one event are deemed to have clinically isolated syndrome. Only time will tell if a patient with clinically isolated syndrome will develop MS.

The formal criteria for diagnosing MS are known as the McDonald Criteria, and they were most recently updated in 2017. It is important to

SUMMARY OF 2017 MCDONALD CRITERIA FOR THE DIAGNOSIS OF MS

✓ *Requires elimination of more likely diagnoses*
✓ *Requires demonstration of dissemination of lesions in the central nervous system in space and time*

CLINICAL PRESENTATION	ADDITIONAL CRITERIA TO MAKE MS DIAGNOSIS
...in a person who has experienced a typical attack/CIS at onset	
• 2 or more attacks and clinical evidence of 2 or more lesions; OR • 2 or more attacks and clinical evidence of 1 lesion with clear historical evidence of prior attack involving lesion in different location	None. DIS and DIT have been met.
• 2 or more attacks and clinical evidence of 1 lesion	DIS shown by <u>one</u> of these criteria: – additional clinical attack implicating different CNS site – 1 or more MS-typical T2 lesions in 2 or more areas of CNS: periventricular, cortical, juxta cortical, infratentorial or spinal cord
• 1 attack and clinical evidence of 2 or more lesions	DIT shown by <u>one</u> of these criteria: – Additional clinical attack – Simultaneous presence of bothenhancing and non-enhancing MS-typical MRI lesions, or new T2 or enhancing MRI lesion compared to baseline scan (without regard to timing of baseline scan) – CSF oligoclonal bands
• 1 attack and clinical evidence of 1: lesion	DIS shown by <u>one</u> of these criteria: – Additional attack implicating different CNS site – I or more MS-typical T2 lesions in 2 or more areas of CNS: periventricular, cortical, juxta cortical, infratentorial or spinal cord **AND** DIT shown by <u>one</u> of these criteria: – additional clinical attack – Simultaneous presence of bothenhancing and non-enhancing MS-typical MRI-lesions, or new T2 or enhancing MRI-lesion compared to baseline scan (without regard to timing of baseline scan) – CSF oligoclonal bands
...in a person who has steady progression of disease since onset	
1 year of disease progression (retrospective or prospective)	DIS shown by at least <u>two</u> of these criteria: – 1 or more MS-typical T2 lesions (periventricular, cortical, juxtacortical or infratentorial) – 2 or more T2 spinal cord lesions – CSF oligoclonal bands

DIT = Dissemination In time   **DIS** = Dissemination in space   **CNS** = Central nervous system
CSF = Cerebrospinal fluid   **T2 lesion** = Hyperintense lesion on T2-weighted MRI

The 2017 McDonald Criteria. (Used with permission of the National Multiple Sclerosis Society.)

remember that these criteria were not delivered to neurologists on stone tablets. Rather, experts in the field meet periodically and decide on these criteria. At some point in the future, they will be tweaked again.

7. Do I Need a Lumbar Puncture?

If an evil doctor wanted to instill fear and horror in the heart of patients everywhere, the doctor would come up with the lumbar puncture. Yet, this is a test that I find myself frequently recommending for some terrified souls. As stated previously, the diagnosis of MS is primarily a clinical one, made by talking to and examining patients. All patients with suspected MS will also have MRIs of their brain and spine. In those patients for whom the history, physical, and MRI are highly suggestive of MS, there is not much of a role for a lumbar puncture.

Approximately 90% of MS patients have a marker of inflammation in the central nervous system called oligoclonal bands. In patients with a single relapse and clinical or MRI demonstration of dissemination in space, the presence of oligoclonal bands allows for a formal diagnosis of MS. Given that most neurologists would suggest treatment to such patients, a lumbar puncture is not always necessary for them either.

However, in ambiguous situations, a lumbar puncture can help determine whether or not the patient has MS. There are some patients for whom the diagnosis of MS is unclear, as many other diseases can mimic MS, both clinically and on the MRI. A lumbar puncture to look for oligoclonal bands is most useful when the history, neurological exam, or MRI are in any way atypical for MS. Examples of atypical presentations include:

- Patients with symptoms not usually seen initially in MS, such as depression, language impairment, or significant cognitive impairment.
- Patients with symptoms that are characteristic of MS, yet with a relatively normal MRI or an MRI that shows abnormalities that are atypical for MS.
- Patients with another illness that can mimic MS.
- Patients outside of the normal age range for MS.
- Patients with symptoms outside of the central nervous system, such as a fever, rash, or weight loss.

If oligoclonal bands are absent in these patients, an alternative diagnosis to MS should be considered. Also, the lumbar puncture should not show too many other abnormalities, such as numerous white blood cells or a very elevated protein level. If these are found, an alternative diagnosis should be sought. Occasionally, some patients request a lumbar puncture, as they want to be as certain as possible about the diagnosis.

The presence or absence of oligoclonal bands may also provide a small clue about the prognosis of MS. One study that investigated the spinal fluid of patients who had a single episode suggestive of MS found that patients with oligoclonal bands had twice the risk for having a second attack, regardless of the initial MRI. The presence of these bands, however, did not seem to influence the development of disability. Another study found that patients with MS, but without oligoclonal bands, "were significantly more likely to exhibit neurological or systemic clinical features atypical of MS (headaches, neuropsychiatric features, and skin changes)." However, other studies have not identified a difference between MS patients with and without oligoclonal bands.

Lastly, oligoclonal bands are not specific for MS, and they can be found in a wide range of other neuro-inflammatory diseases.

8.   *What Should I Expect With a Lumbar Puncture?*

WILL IT HURT? It might. Lumbar punctures require placing a needle into the back. A local anesthetic will be applied to numb the area, but most people can expect some degree of pain. In my hospital, we are spoiled in having radiologists perform the lumbar punctures. They are able to use imaging to guide the needle right where it needs to go. In most cases, however, the lumbar puncture is performed at the bedside by a neurologist who guides the needle by feeling alone. Naturally, the ease of this procedure depends on the experience of the neurologist and the size of the person undergoing the lumbar puncture.

In my experience, patients vary widely in their tolerance of lumbar punctures. I had one patient fall asleep during what is usually the most painful part, while others have screamed in pain when I washed their back. If someone is terrified, a mild sedative may help.

Some patients develop a headache a day or two after a lumbar puncture. This headache, while not serious, can be very painful. It is a positional headache that lessens when people lie down but returns with a vengeance when they stand up. Fortunately, there is a simple cure for this called a blood patch. In a blood patch, a doctor will inject the patient's own blood at the same location as the original lumbar puncture. This procedure is highly effective in instantly and permanently eliminating the headache.

IS IT DANGEROUS? Not really. When done properly, there is very little risk for any serious complication, such as paralysis or infection. The procedure does have to be done in a sterile fashion to minimize the risk of infection. This does not mean that it has to be done in a sterile operating room, however. To minimize the risk of bleeding, a lumbar puncture should not be performed on someone with a bleeding disorder.

Fortunately, a lumbar puncture is a procedure that someone with a possible diagnosis of MS needs only experience once. It usually takes about 30 minutes, and patients can leave as soon as it is over, though they are advised to relax for the rest of the day. So, while it can be painful and scary, it should not be viewed as a "major procedure" or something that carries a significant risk of permanent damage.

In summary, a lumbar puncture is most useful in patients for whom the clinical diagnosis of MS is a possibility, but not a certainty. Although it is unpleasant to undergo a lumbar puncture, it is worth doing in some patients, given that it might make the difference between a diagnosis of MS or not.

9. What Are the Initial Symptoms of MS?

Since MS can affect the entire brain and spinal cord, the initial symptoms of MS can include almost any symptom in neurology. However, some symptoms are more common than others. Weakness and sensory disturbances are the two most common initial symptoms in MS, simply because these axons span the length of the central nervous system, from the surface of the brain to the end of the spinal cord. Any MS lesion is, therefore, very likely to affect one or both of these pathways. Visual symptoms—a painful, partial loss of vision in one eye (termed optic neuritis), or double vision—are also very common initial symptoms. The symptoms usually do not develop suddenly, like a stroke, but come on over the course of several hours or days.

The most common initial symptoms in MS are:

- Sensory abnormalities (occurs in 34% of people with MS), which is a numbness and tingling in the feet, hands, torso, or one side of the face
- Weakness (22%)
- Visual loss or double vision (21%)
- Clumsiness (11%)
- Vertigo (4%)

Other characteristic symptoms include Lhermitte's sign, which is a brief shock-like sensation that some patients have when they flex their neck due to a lesion in the cervical spine. Other patients may have an unpleasant squeezing sensation on their torso, which is informally termed the "MS hug."

It is often easy for people to ignore a little numbness or weakness, especially as these symptoms often go away without any treatment. It is also common for doctors to misattribute the initial symptoms of MS to something more benign, such as a "pinched nerve" or muscle strain. Occasionally, a patient will have MS for many years before they seek medical attention or receive the correct diagnosis. In contrast, symptoms such as visual loss, double vision, imbalance, and vertigo are less likely to be ignored or misdiagnosed. Other neurological symptoms, such as cognitive deficits, psychiatric symptoms, and language difficulties, may be the initial symptom of MS, but this is extremely rare.

10. *What Is a Relapse?*

Relapses, which are also called flares, attacks, or exacerbations, are a hallmark feature of MS. This characteristic defines the disease for most people, at least in the early stages, and most of the medicines for MS have been approved based on their ability to prevent relapses. Despite this, some patients are confused about what a relapse actually is and what it means for their prognosis.

Let me clarify some important points in the definition of a relapse based on conversations I have had with patients who are confused by this admittedly confusing topic.

First of all, relapses have to last at least 24 hours, although usually they last at least several days or weeks. I have met many worried patients who believe they have had numerous relapses after experiencing a transient neurological symptom lasting for only a few minutes. With rare exceptions

What Is a Relapse?

- Neurological disturbance of kind seen in MS.
- Subjective report or objective observation.
- At least 24 hours duration in absence of fever or infection.
- Excludes pseudoattacks, single paroxysmal symptoms (multiple episodes of paroxysmal symptoms occurring over 24 hours or more are acceptable as evidence.)
- Some historical events with symptoms and pattern typical for MS can provide reasonable evidence of previous demyelinating event(s), even without objective findings.

Determining Time Between Attacks

- At least 30 days between onset of event 1 and 2

(such as pain on one side of the face), these transient events are not considered relapses. Persistent symptoms of fatigue or "brain fog" are also not considered relapses, though they can be quite disabling.

Also, to be considered a relapse, the symptom almost always has to be something brand new. Many patients recover well from relapses, though sometimes the recovery is not complete. Symptoms such as tingling, weakness, stiffness, visual loss, or double vision may come and go for reasons that are not entirely clear. These fluctuations of existing symptoms are not considered to be relapses. Admittedly, it is often difficult to tell if a patient is having a new relapse or a recurrence of an old symptom.

Moreover, a relapse cannot occur in the setting of a fever or infection. When the symptoms of a relapse occur in these circumstances, it is termed a *pseudorelapse*. During a pseudorelapse, patients can feel worse, but this usually is due to the re-emergence of old, partially healed symptoms when the body is stressed. This most commonly occurs in the setting of a urinary tract infection. Fatigue or stress may also bring out old symptoms.

To understand why pseudorelapses may occur, consider the scenario of a broken bone. Though a bone may heal, it will probably not return to its full strength. If it is stressed again, it is more likely to break in the same location. The same is true in MS and for the nervous system; fevers, infections, or metabolic derangements can cause old, previously healed, symptoms to temporarily return. This is why many neurologists will inquire about symptoms of an infection and check for a urinary tract infection prior to treating patients for a relapse. It is important that patients tell their neurologist about any symptoms of an infection if they feel they are experiencing a relapse.

11.   What Are the Stages and Different Types of MS?

MS presents in very different ways in different patients, and several different categories have been defined. The most common way to categorize MS, however, is to track its course over time. At present, there are four categories of MS:

CATEGORY 1: CLINICALLY ISOLATED SYNDROME (CIS): Patients who have had one clinical event are said to have clinically isolated syndrome or CIS. If certain findings are present on either the MRI or in the cerebrospinal fluid, patients with one clinical event can be diagnosed with MS. Otherwise, a diagnosis of MS can be made only if the patient develops lesions not previously seen on the MRI or experiences a second clinical event. The distinction between MS and CIS is somewhat artificial. CIS is usually a precursor to MS, not a different disease. Because the evidence suggests that MS is best treated in its early stages, most neurologists recommend initiating treatment after the first event indicative of MS.

CATEGORY 2: RELAPSING-REMITTING MS (RRMS): About 90 percent of patients are diagnosed with relapsing-remitting MS (RRMS). This term refers to the tendency of an MS symptom to develop rather abruptly (a relapse) and to then gradually abate over the next few days or weeks (a remission). Usually patients recover well, but it is common to be left with some residual symptoms. There can be a high degree of variability in the specific symptoms, the frequency, the severity, and the degree of recovery from relapses. But as long as patients are experiencing relapses without progression of their symptoms in between, they are considered to have RRMS.

RRMS is further subdivided as follows:

- **Active:** The patient is experiencing a relapse and/or new MRI activity.

- **Not active:** No disease activity is occurring.

- **Not active but worsening:** Disability becomes worse as symptoms persist.

- **Active but not worsening:** There is new MRI activity, but no worsening of disability or new clinical symptoms.

Almost all of the treatments available for MS have been studied and approved for RRMS. Therefore, it is very important that neurologists spend time talking with their patients to understand not only their current symptoms, but how these symptoms began and progressed over time.

CATEGORY 3: SECONDARY PROGRESSIVE MS (SPMS): After 15 to 20, years most patients with RRMS enter what is called the secondary-progressive phase (SPMS). In SPMS, relapses either disappear completely or are very infrequent. Yet there is a slow but steady increase in disability. Patients in this stage of the illness may tell you that 1 year ago they could walk 10 blocks before needing a rest, but now they can walk only eight. Patients with SPMS develop symptoms similar to the way my hair is going gray, slowly but surely.

There is no formal transition between RRMS and SPMS, nor are there laboratory tests or radiographic tests to distinguish between these two stages of the illness. Again, the SPMS stage of the illness can only be determined by talking with patients to understand their current symptoms and examining them. Patients who are diagnosed at a younger age tend to remain in the RRMS phase longer than those who are diagnosed at a later age.

Unfortunately, most disability accumulates in the SPMS phase, and this is where treatments are currently lacking. As with RRMS, however, there is a large range of disability experienced by patients with SPMS. Most patients fear the SPMS stage the most, anticipating a gradual, inevitable decline in their ability to function. However, aside from the inevitable decline associated with aging, a fair number of patients with SPMS experience little or no progression during the later stages of the disease.

CATEGORY 4: PRIMARY PROGRESSIVE MS (PPMS): About 10% of patients present with a progressive form of MS at onset without relapses. This is known as primary progressive MS (PPMS). It is characterized by steadily worsening neurological function or disability from the onset of symptoms. To diagnose PPMS, there must be 1 year of disease progression. Unlike RRMS, PPMS presents equally in men and women, and tends to occur at an older age. It almost always presents with gradual trouble walking. Certain presentations, such as optic neuritis, that are common in RRMS are rare in PPMS. Enhancing MRI lesions indicative of active inflammation are also less common in PPMS than RRMS. PPMS patients usually accumulate disability more rapidly than patients with RRMS.

A diagnosis of PPMS may be further modified at any point in time as:

■ **Active**: With new MRI activity and/or relapses and/or new lesions on the MRI.

■ **Not active**: Without new MRI activity and/or relapses.

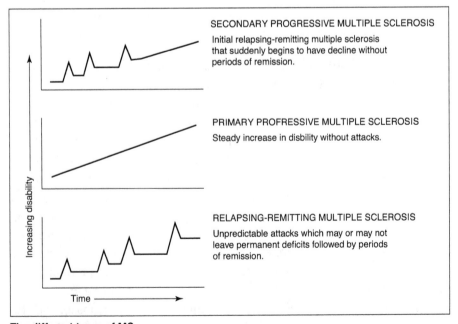

The different types of MS.

In addition, both active and not active PPMS may be further modified as:

▓ **With progression:** There is objective evidence of increased disability

▓ **Without progression:** There is no objective evidence of increased disability

Lastly, some patients may be diagnosed with an entity called radiographically isolated syndrome (RIS). RIS occurs when a patient gets an MRI because of a non-MS symptom (such as a headache), but the MRI reveals lesions that are characteristic for MS. One of my patients got an MRI after getting into a car crash, and it looked utterly classic for MS. Although there is some disagreement, most neurologists would suggest treating such patients with medications to hopefully prevent symptoms and disability in the future.

12.   How Can I Tell What Stage of MS I'm in?

A natural question is whether patients are in the relapsing remitting phase (RRMS), secondary progressive phase (SPMS), or progressive phase (PPMS). Let's again review what these terms mean. About 90% of patients start with RRMS. This means that they develop a neurological symptom, usually over the course of hours to days, which then spontaneously improves over days to weeks. The recovery from relapses is usually quite good, though this is not always the case. Patients may then go months to years before they have another relapse, and there is no or minimal development of disability in between relapses. After 15 to 20 years, patients will then enter the SPMS. Relapses are very rare or absent in SPMS. However, patients may accumulate gradual disability from year to year.

Often it is quite clear when patients are in the RRMS or the SPMS phase of the illness, but there is no formal transition between the two stages. In this way, it can be compared to asking "when does someone become old?" A person who lives to 100 is old by any definition, but no one can tell you the exact moment they became "old."

Though it is not always easy, it is important to determine the stage of a patient's MS to the best of our abilities. The treatments are most effective with RRMS and are of minimal benefit in SPMS. One of the challenges faced by neurologists and patients alike is to be bold enough to stop using medications for MS in patients who are clearly in the PPMS phase and for whom relapses are no longer a concern.

Finally, the divisions of MS into RRMS and SPMS say nothing about the disease severity or what symptoms are present. Some patients have very mild progressive MS, while others have severe RRMS. In this sense, one stage of the illness is not "better" than another.

13. What Is the Prognosis of MS?

MS is a disease that causes a very wide spectrum of symptoms and disability. A natural question asked by a newly diagnosed patient is, "What is going to happen to me?" For some patients, MS will be little more than a mild nuisance. Many patients will live full, complete lives. There are some people who, unfortunately, will suffer life-altering disability at an early age. Generally speaking, about one third of patients will have minimal disease that impairs only the most vigorous activities; one third will have moderate disease; and one third will have more severe disease that prevents them from working or living independently. It is my hope that we are able to improve these numbers with new, effective treatments.

The wide range of symptoms and disability among MS patients makes it challenging to provide more than a general prognosis, especially early in the course of the disease. However, some prognostic factors have been discovered. Following an MS diagnosis, favorable prognostic factors include:

- Caucasian race
- Female sex
- Younger age at disease onset
- Sensory symptoms at onset
- Full recovery from the initial relapse
- Fewer relapses in the years after diagnosis
- Fewer lesions on the baseline MRI

Keep in mind these are generalizations and can only give a rough estimate of disease severity over time. Each individual case follows its own unique course. As with all generalizations, they will not apply to all individuals. For example, men are usually taller than women, but this is certainly not always the case.

The same is true with MS. I know young, White females who have had a very difficult time. I also know older African American males who have little clinical evidence of the disease. Additionally, the prognostic factors can sometimes be misleading. Even though younger patients generally have slower progression of their symptoms, they are going to live longer and will have more time to develop additional or worsening symptoms.

If I could add any tool to my treatment arsenal for patients with MS (other than a cure), it would be a crystal ball. Some patients are destined to have mild disease even without treatment. My aunt, for example, had a very clear episode suggestive of MS when she was 30 years old. She is now 80, still working, and outlasted me during a recent hike. At present, we cannot predict early on who those relatively fortunate patients are. As a result, most neurologists suggest the initiation of early treatment, even in those patients who do not meet the formal criteria for MS. When these patients do well, we can never know for certain if it is because the medication is working or because they were destined to have mild disease.

Unfortunately, there are also young patients who are going to have a severe disease, and we often cannot predict who these patients will be early in the disease course. Several years ago, when there were fewer treatments available to patients, predicting a patient's clinical course would have limited value. However, with the approval of powerful medicines to treat MS, the issue of prognosis has grown in importance. Hopefully, future research will provide better tools to give more accurate prognoses for MS. The hope is that we will be able to recognize which patients should be started on aggressive therapy and which patients might never need treatment at all.

14. What Is the Life Expectancy for People With MS?

Several studies have examined the life expectancy of people with MS. One review found that people with MS live 7 to 14 years less compared to people without MS. Another study of over 30,000 patients found that people with MS live an average of 6 years less. While this may seem discouraging, the majority of patients will lead full, long lives. Unfortunately, a small number of patients will become bedbound. These patients are at risk for complications that shorten life expectancy, bringing down the average for the entire group of MS patients. To consider how extremes can affect an average value, consider Bill Gates going to a homeless shelter. By averaging, his wealth would make it appear as if every person there was a millionaire. It should also be noted that MS itself is almost never directly fatal. I have never seen a patient die from an MS relapse.

15. Will I Wake up One Day and Not Be Able to Walk?

The short answer to this question, is almost always "NO!" Many patients naturally wonder if they are likely to be significantly and permanently disabled from a relapse. They are understandably fearful that they will wake up one morning unable to walk or suffer some other severe disability.

MS patients should know that a single relapse is unlikely to be a permanently devastating event. On the other hand, just because a patient is not experiencing relapses, this does not mean that they are disease free. The current thinking about MS is that it is both an *inflammatory* disorder, where the inflammation manifests as relapses, and a *neurodegenerative* disorder (like Alzheimer's or Parkinson's disease), where there is a slow, steady progression of symptoms over years and decades. The inflammatory part of MS predominates early on, while the degenerative process is a later feature. Unfortunately, much of the disability from MS occurs in the progressive phase, and our ability to slow down progression is limited at present.

16. Do Relapses Matter?

If most of the disability occurs in the progressive phase, does this mean that relapses don't matter? Since the main MS medications are used to prevent relapses, are we tricking ourselves into thinking that we are having an impact on the course of the disease? Several well-respected neurologists have written that relapses really don't significantly impact long-term disability. After all, about 10% of patients have primary progressive MS (PPMS). These patients do not have relapses yet they generally accumulate disability at a faster rate than patients with relapsing remitting MS (RRMS).

Despite this, I believe that relapses matter, even though they are not likely to be permanently devastating events and much of disability increases during the progressive phase. Firstly, even if relapses have minimal effect on patients' long-term physical disability, they can cause significant emotional distress. I have seen many patients who are having what might appear to be a "minor" relapse pay a significant emotional price, knowing that their disease is not under control.

Secondly, the studies I discussed used the Expanded Disability Status Scale (EDSS) to measure disability, as do most studies in MS. I will discuss it more later, but briefly, the EDSS is a scale that is heavily dependent on a patient's ability to walk. However, I have seen patients suffer relapses characterized by pain, visual difficulties, and cognitive disturbances. Who can argue that these symptoms do not matter? Yet, based on the EDSS, these patients might not be considered as having significant disability, as long as their ability to walk was not affected.

Finally, while the prevention of long-term disability is what most neurologists and patients care about, the short-term should not be undervalued. It is very common for patients who have relapses to be left with abnormal sensations, weakness, visual disturbances, and other symptoms. While these symptoms may not make a difference in how someone is doing 20 years after a relapse, they can make a huge difference in how someone is doing 20 days after a relapse. Why should this not matter?

What does this mean in terms of treating MS? If a medication were invented tomorrow that completely eliminated relapses, it is doubtful that MS would be cured. Yet, there is evidence that, over periods lasting several years, patients who take medicines for MS have less disability than those given placebo in the clinical trials, indicating to me that relapse prevention in MS is no trivial matter. I prescribe medications for MS patients with confidence that they have a positive influence on the course of the illness, while at the same time recognizing there is much work to be done before the disease can be conquered.

17.   *What About Pediatric MS?*

MS typically affects young and middle-aged adults, but about 3% of patients develop symptoms during childhood or adolescence. Pediatric MS is defined as MS occurring in children under 18 years of age. Most patients with pediatric MS are adolescents. Only very rarely do symptoms present before age 10 years.

Pediatric MS is the same condition as adult MS. Usually the symptoms and laboratory and MRI findings are similar to adults with MS. Like adults, children present with several days or weeks of vision loss, sensory disturbances, weakness, or balance problems that tend to improve, usually back to normal.

There are some differences, however. Relapses tend to occur more frequently in children than adults, but children recover more quickly and more fully from relapses than adults. Importantly, children always present with RRMS. PPMS does not occur in children. So, children who experience years of struggling in school and notice that their problems are getting worse do not have MS.

Increasingly, MS centers are gaining experience helping children. A number of centers have been specifically established for pediatric MS in the United States and around the world. They are working together to help ensure that children get the best possible care.

2 THE MRI AND MS

18. What Is an MRI and What Does It Show in MS?

Magnetic resonance image (MRI) scans of the brain and spinal cord area are a frequent part of life for many MS patients. As the name implies, an MRI is a powerful magnet that gives an amazing view into the structures of the central nervous system. By administering a contrast agent called gadolinium, areas of active inflammation can be detected. Unlike computed tomography or CT or CAT scans, MRIs do not use radiation. So, unless patients are allergic to the contrast agent or have metal in their bodies, MRI scans are entirely safe. MRIs take about 1 to 2 hours to perform, and some patients need a mild sedative if they are claustrophobic.

Most of the MRI lesions (also called plaques) in MS can be likened to scars in that they represent areas of old injury. Although they can regress over time, usually once a lesion is present, it rarely goes away entirely. As with an old scar, an old lesion does not necessarily cause symptoms. Lesions that become bright with the administration of contrast agent represent active areas of inflammation. They are more common in the earlier stages of MS and are the radiographic correlate of a relapse. Prevention of MRI lesions is a major outcome in clinical trials, though the exact degree to which MRI lesions correlate with a patient's clinical outcome is somewhat controversial.

19. How Are MRIs Used to Diagnose MS?

As previously discussed, the diagnosis of MS requires demonstrated inflammation in different parts of the central nervous system (this is referred to as dissemination in space) and at different points of time (this is referred to as dissemination in time). Historically, an MS diagnosis relied solely on a patient's history and physical examination. While the history and exam are still the best way to diagnose MS, the modern diagnostic criteria allow MRI abnormalities to replace clinical symptoms and exam abnormalities.

Formal criteria have been established so that the MRI can be used to show the dissemination in time and space, allowing doctors to diagnose MS in patients who have had only one clinical event. These formal MRI criteria for diagnosis follow.

DISSEMINATION IN TIME:
- A single MRI showing both a lesion that enhances with contrast (indicating active inflammation) as well as non-enhancing lesions, indicating prior inflammation.
- A new lesion on any follow-up MRI done after the original image.

DISSEMINATION IN SPACE:
- More than one lesion in at least two out of four areas of the central nervous system: periventricular, juxtacortical, infratentorial, or the spinal cord. Examples of these lesions follow.

Let's examine what this all means along with the different kinds of MRIs used in MS. Most typically, MS appears as oval-shaped white lesions (informally called Dawson's fingers) that radiate away from the ventricles, which are the fluid-filled spaces in the center of the brain. These are called periventricular lesions.

Lesions adjacent to the grey matter in the cerebral cortex are called juxtacortical lesions. They are near the brain's surface but are still in the white matter. Lesions in lower parts of the brain, namely the brainstem and cerebellum, are called infratentorial lesions. Lastly, lesions can appear

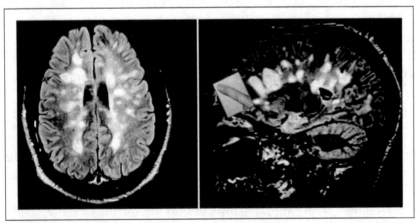

MRIs demonstrating oval-shaped, white lesions near the ventricles, which are called Dawson's fingers, which are very characteristic of MS. The right-hand picture includes an image of a finger to illustrate the similarity.

throughout the thoracic and cervical spine. These lesions are often symptomatic, causing weakness and sensory disturbances. For every clinic event a patient feels, the MRI will generally show 5 to 10 times as many lesions. Usually, by the time a patient experiences their first symptom, the MRI shows several lesions indicating the patient likely has had the illness for some time. Although it is technically possible for patients with MS to have a normal MRI, few neurologists would feel comfortable diagnosing the disease if there were no lesions at all.

One of strongest correlations between how a patient is doing clinically and their MRI are areas where both the axons and the myelin have been injured. These dark lesions are called "black holes." They may take months or years to develop and are often not seen in newly diagnosed patients. If they are present in newly diagnosed patients, it is evidence that they have had the disease for some time without clinical symptoms.

In longstanding MS, there may be generalized brain atrophy. The following image shows an enlargement of the ventricles. Atrophy most likely manifests as cognitive impairment rather than a focal neurological symptom. Although sophisticated measures can show evidence of brain atrophy in early MS, it usually becomes obvious only after several decades. Even then, it is not obvious in many patients.

Rarely, patients will present with a large area of demyelination referred to as a tumefactive lesion. Such patients may present with language

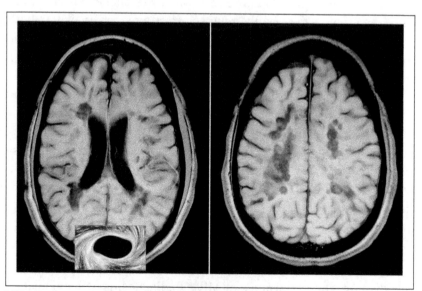

MRIs demonstrating multiple "black holes" in a patient with longstanding MS.

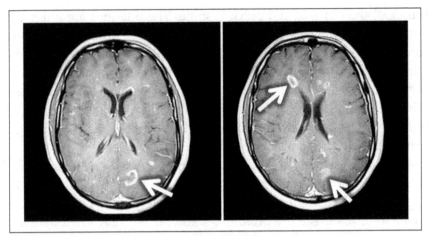

MRIs demonstrating numerous enhancing lesions, including solid, ring, and horseshoe lesions.

disturbances, visual field deficits, cognitive and personality changes, or severe weakness and sensory loss on one side of the body. Both the clinical presentation and the radiographic appearance of the lesions can mimic a tumor or infection. On rare occasions, a biopsy may be needed before the correct diagnosis is made.

20.   How Do MRIs Help With Relapses?

In addition to helping to diagnose MS, MRIs are also essential whenever patients experience a possible relapse. In almost every MRI, patients receive a contrast agent called gadolinium. It normally stays in the blood-stream and does not enter the brain. If there is a breakdown in the barrier between the brain and its blood vessels, the dye can enter the central ner-vous system and appear bright on the MRI. This is called enhancement, and in MS it means there is active inflammation.

Enhancing lesions in MS appear either solid, ring shaped, or horseshoe shaped. Enhancement can occur in any part of the central nervous system, including the brain, brainstem, cerebellum, and the spinal cord.

Nearly all relapses are associated with contrast-enhancing lesions. Additionally, MRIs may reveal enhancing lesions in patients without new symptoms.

21.   How Do MRIs Help With Disease Surveillance?

No one disputes the importance of MRIs in diagnosing MS and evaluating patients for relapses. Once the diagnosis of MS has been made, however, the role of the MRI is somewhat murkier, at least in patients who are clinically stable. Many patients view the MRI as a crystal ball into their future. I discourage this way of thinking. I have seen patients who have been clinically stable for many years become terrified upon learning their MRI shows a single new lesion. Though MRIs are visually compelling, and no one wants to hear "you have a new lesion in your brain," the MRI is not a perfect indicator of how a patient is actually doing. Some patients have MRIs that reveal numerous lesions though they feel fine and their exams are nearly normal. In contrast, other patients have minimal changes on their MRI, but suffer more disability. This mismatch between how a patient feels and how the MRI looks is referred to as the "clinical-radiographical paradox." Of course, how patients feel matters much more than the findings on their MRIs.

Having said this, new MRI lesions matter even if patients don't feel them. So-called "silent lesions" are not harmless and should not be ignored. Patients who do not feel a new lesion are at risk for developing one that they will feel. Additionally, multiple asymptomatic lesions may become symptomatic over time. Fatigue and cognitive impairment are likely due in part to the accumulation of "silent lesions" over many years. It's possible also that if detailed cognitive tests were carried out, these so-called "silent lesions" would not be silent after all. About 70% of lesions are "silent," especially in the brain. In contrast, most lesions in the spinal cord cause symptoms.

Given this, most neurologists order MRIs of the brain every 6 to 12 months to see if new lesions are developing in the absence of clinical symptoms. This is especially important in younger, newly diagnosed patients and less valuable in older, stable patients who have had the disease for many years. While there is some variation, most neurologists would agree that patients who develop multiple, silent lesions in a short period of time are in danger of having a relapse and worsening disability. As such, most neurologists feel it is appropriate to change therapies rather than wait until someone has a clinical relapse. Though I try to treat the human sitting in front of me rather than the MRI on the screen, in many cases of silent lesions, I will change a patient's medication to hopefully prevent new lesions and, more importantly, new symptoms.

22. Do All White Spots Mean MS?

It is important to note that not all white spots mean MS. The MRI is an extraordinarily powerful tool. Its ability to allow us to see the brain is comparable to a dermatologist using a magnifying glass to conduct a skin exam. Even in completely healthy people, *something* abnormal will be found on their skin. No one has blemish-free skin.

The same problem occurs with MRIs. As one doctor said, "It is very rare for an MRI to come back with the words 'normal study.' I can't tell you the last time I've seen it." Unfortunately, MRIs often detect lesions that are of no clinical significance, and these abnormalities can easily be mistaken for the lesions of MS. In fact, white matter lesions in the brain are so common that radiologists informally call them "unidentified bright objects" or UBOs. UBOs are more common in older people, especially if they smoked or have diseases such as hypertension, migraines, or diabetes. Sometimes, even young patients have many UBOs, and we are not sure why. When confronted with this picture, many radiologists will give a long list of possibilities that the lesions *could* be. Many patients are naturally frightened when the radiologist's report says that these lesions could be "ischemic, infectious, vasculitis, demyelinating, or due to migraine."

So how should neurologists handle such cases? We pride ourselves on being perhaps the last type of doctor who believe the best way to evaluate patients is to talk to them and examine them. Yes, the MRI is incredibly valuable in MS. However, MRI abnormalities must be interpreted in the proper clinical context. An MRI does not take the place of a careful history and physical examination.

Occasionally, I have met patients who have been improperly diagnosed with MS, I believe, and have taken burdensome medicines and lived with a worrisome diagnosis for many years largely because of a few white dots on their MRI. In fact, the over-diagnosis of MS is almost certainly a bigger problem than the under-diagnosis of MS. At times I have to "take away" a diagnosis of MS. Understandably, this can be very upsetting for patients. Other times, I have diagnosed rare conditions that can mimic MS. Patients who feel they have been misdiagnosed with MS should not hesitate to seek a second opinion.

3 TREATING MS PART I: RELAPSES

The treatment of MS includes treating relapses, preventing relapses and disability, and minimizing symptoms. It involves medications, procedures, devices, physical and occupational therapy, nursing care, social work, psychotherapy, and support from family and friends.

23.   How Are Relapses Treated?

In almost all cases, relapses are treated with high doses of steroids. This is one of the oldest, most well-established treatments in MS. Steroids are naturally occurring compounds made by the adrenal glands. Steroids are usually quite effective in speeding up the rate at which a patient improves after a relapse. There is not much evidence that steroids have a long-term impact on the course of MS, however. In a study of patients with optic neuritis (pain and temporary vision loss) as a first presentation of possible MS, patients treated with steroids had a lower rate of conversion to clinically definite MS. However, there was no overall difference in visual acuity between patients who received steroids and those who did not.

There are several different types of steroids, but the most commonly used steroid in MS is Solu-Medrol (methylprednisolone). It is usually given intravenously (IV) for 3 to 5 days, but occasionally is given for longer periods if the relapse is severe. Patients do not have to enter the hospital if they have access to an infusion center. In some cases, it can be given at a patient's home by a visiting nurse.

There is evidence that oral steroids are as effective as IV steroids, though patients will have to take over 20 pills a day to reach the same dose as the IV steroids. Additionally, oral steroids have more gastrointestinal side effects than IV steroids.

Some patients report a significant "boost" from steroids, even without a new relapse. For these patients, steroids are sometimes given on a schedule as infrequently as twice per year. This protocol is called "pulse steroids." However, there is no evidence that pulse steroids have any long-term impact in preventing future relapses or on the long-term progression of the disease.

24.   What Are the Side Effects of Steroids?

Unfortunately, steroids can have some unpleasant side effects. For the short courses given in MS, steroids are almost always well-tolerated. The most common side effects are psychiatric; some patients become depressed. At other times, patients become manic and even psychotic. For this reason, many patients take a small dose of a mild sedative called Klonopin (clonazepam) while on steroids. Other side effects include temporary weight gain and an upset stomach, so most patients will take an antacid to prevent peptic ulcers. Patients with diabetes can have elevated blood sugars and may need to be admitted to the hospital for closer monitoring. The same can be true for patients with hypertension. Some patients request a steroid taper to help minimize the side effects of abruptly stopping high-dose steroids.

Over the long term, steroids can cause even more side effects including cataracts, bone destruction, gastric ulcers, diabetes, and significant weight gain. For this reason, steroids cannot be given on a continuous basis.

25.   Are There Options Besides Steroids for Relapses?

In certain patients, steroids are not an option. Either they have poor venous access, or they cannot tolerate their side effects, or the steroids failed to relieve the symptoms of their relapse.

26.   What Is Acthar?

Another option to treat relapses is adrenocorticotropic hormone (ACTH), called Acthar gel. ACTH is a naturally occurring hormone that stimulates the adrenal glands to make several different steroid hormones. It is given as an intramuscular injection at full dose for a week, then at a lower dose for several weeks afterward. Patients are instructed how to give the injections themselves. Acthar is as effective as steroids and may have fewer side effects, though overall its side effects are similar to steroids. The main disadvantage is its cost. Because it is very expensive, insurance companies can take several days to approve Acthar. It is, therefore, not an ideal option for patients who need immediate treatment.

27.   What Is Plasmapheresis?

A procedure called plasmapheresis is an option for patients who have a significant relapse that does not respond to steroids. In this procedure, a large IV line is placed, and the patient's blood is then filtered through a machine that separates the blood cells from other components in the bloodstream. Plasmapheresis usually requires 7 to 10 days in the hospital, and each treatment takes several hours. Some patients may be able to get this treatment as an outpatient.

There are some risks to the procedure. The placement of the catheter itself carries a low risk for infection and a collapsed lung. Prior to each treatment, blood tests have to be done to make sure that there are no deficits of the blood's coagulation proteins. Nonetheless, I have seen several patients who have had relapses that were unresponsive to steroids improve significantly after a course of plasmapheresis. It is certainly worth trying in patients with significant relapses that are not alleviated by steroids.

Of course, physical and occupational therapy are invaluable throughout the course of MS. However, they may be more important after a relapse to maximize the degree and rate of recovery.

4 TREATING MS PART II: DISEASE-MODIFYING THERAPIES

28. What Are the Disease-Modifying Therapies?

The first treatment for MS, an injectable interferon medicine called interferon-beta (Betaseron), was approved by the FDA in 1993. Historically, the first-line treatments for MS patients were interferons or Copaxone, another injectable medication. These medicines have been used by hundreds of thousands of people over 25 years and have a very strong track record in terms of both safety and efficacy. However, they are far from a cure and have potentially intolerable side effects. In recent years, more effective therapies, including three oral medications and several infusible medications have been approved. Several more are likely to emerge in the near future. It is hard to think of a field of medicine that has changed more in the past decade than MS.

Nothing is for free, however, and with these more powerful treatments come more powerful side effects. When evaluating a medication, we must try to balance the risks versus the benefits. In determining which medication to suggest, what we are trying to do is determine what we fear more—the disease or the medication. For patients who seem to have mild MS, treating them with a powerful but potentially dangerous medication would be inappropriate. One obvious rule of thumb is that a medication should never cause more problems than it solves. Similarly, in patients who seem to have aggressive disease, treating them with a safe but less effective medication would not be wise.

As I write this, there are over a dozen medications available, each with their own risk/benefit profile. This is good news, of course, but these choices can pose a challenge for both neurologists and patients. Too many choices can be overwhelming. Choosing a medication can be like going to a diner with a 20-page menu.

Often patients anguish and debate about which medicine to start taking. This is understandable but unnecessary, I believe. While the decision about which medicine to choose is certainly an important decision, it is not a major decision, in my opinion, simply because it is so easy to reverse. If a patient has a problem with one medication, with a few exceptions, it is a simple matter to switch to another one. Obviously, neurologists want patients to do well with their first medication. We hope that patients will tolerate it and that it will control their MS. However, choosing a medication is not like getting a tattoo or undergoing a major operation. Changing medications is almost always a simple matter. Only in the most extreme cases is there a need to get it "right" the first time.

The decision about which medication to start is a collaboration between patients and their neurologists. Ultimately, it is a patient's choice which medication to take. However, it is a neurologist's job to give patients recommendations. It is fair for patients to ask their neurologist "Which medication do you think I should take?" Most often, there is no single "right" answer. Patients differ in their tolerance for risk, and neurologists will not always agree on the appropriate treatment. It is my practice to let patients choose which medication to start, though I am not obligated to prescribe a medication if I feel it is unsafe. Also, I certainly will choose a medication when patients ask me to do so.

29. How Do We Evaluate the Medications for MS?

The gold standard to evaluate a medicine is randomized, double-blind, clinical trials. *Randomization* means that study subjects are randomly assigned to receive the study medication or not. In most studies, the study medication is compared to an inert placebo, while other trials use an established MS medication. However, patients are not allowed to choose which treatment they receive. In *double-blind* studies, neither the patient nor the researcher knows which treatment anyone received until the trial ends. Randomization and blinding allows us to better determine if a medication truly works or not.

Most studies last 1 to 3 years and enroll approximately 1,000 subjects. Subjects are usually between the ages of 18 and 55 and are healthy other than their MS. Trials enroll patients at MS centers from all over the world. Most medications have several trials that demonstrate their safety and efficacy before they are approved by the FDA.

In judging a medication's benefits, the most commonly used outcome measures are whether the medication lowers the relapse rate and disability progression. All trials also study whether the medication prevents new

MRI lesions. These outcomes are sometimes bunched together in a metric called No Evidence of Disease Activity (NEDA). NEDA occurs in patients who have no relapses, no disability progression, and no new MRI lesions.

The risks of the medication are also carefully studied in clinical trials. When evaluating a medication's side effects, we must consider both tolerability and safety. *Tolerability* refers to side effects such as upset stomach or hair loss. These side effects aren't "serious," but can obviously make life unpleasant. *Safety* refers to potentially serious side effects. Let me be blunt: Some of the MS medications have severely disabled or killed patients.

Lastly, many rare side effects don't emerge in clinical trials, which are relatively short in duration and don't enroll tens of thousands of patients. For this reason, the drug manufacturers do their best to keep track of medications after they have been approved for the general public. This system seems to be working. Neurologists are provided with regular safety updates for many of the medications. In extreme circumstances, a medication may be taken off the market. For example, in March of 2018, a medication called Zinbryta (daclizumab) was removed after some patients developed liver damage and other patients developed encephalitis.

30.   What Is the EDSS?

The Expanded Disability Status Scale (EDSS), mentioned earlier, is the most commonly used rating scale to evaluate patients with MS. It is a standard outcome measure in clinical trials. It measures disability along seven separate parameters: strength, sensation, brainstem functions (eye movements, speech, and swallowing), coordination, vision, cognition, and bowel/bladder continence. It has the advantage of being a well-accepted measure of disability and is not particularly difficult or time consuming to perform.

The EDSS is a 10-point scale that can essentially be divided into three sections:

- **Scores 1–4:** Patients unrestricted in their walking but may have significant disability in other areas.

- **Scores 4–7:** Patients are unable to walk without the use of assistive devices.

- **Scores 7–10:** Patients are bed-bound and may require near-total care.

The Expanded Disability Status Scale

0.0: Normal Neurological Exam

1.0: No disability, minimal signs in 1 FS

1.5: No disability, minimal signs in more than 1 FS

2.0: Minimal disability in 1 FS

2.5: Mild disability in 1 or Minimal disability in 2 FS

3.0: Moderate disability in 1 FS or mild disability in 3–4 FS, though fully ambulatory

3.5: Fully ambulatory but with moderate disability in 1 FS and mild disability in 1 or 2 FS; or moderate disability in 2 FS; or mild disability in 5 FS

4.0: Fully ambulatory without aid, up and about 12hrs a day despite relatively severe disability. Able to walk without a id 500 meters

4.5: Fully ambulatory without a id, up and about much of day, able to work a full day, may otherwise have some limitations of full activity or require minimal assistance. Relatively severe disability. Able to walk without aid 300 meters

5.0: Ambulatory without aid for about 200 meters. Disability impairs full daily activities

5.5: Ambulatory for 100 meters, disability precludes full daily activities

6.0: Intermittent or unilateral constant assistance (cane, crutch or brace) required to walk 100 meters with or without resting

6.5: Constant bilateral support (cane, crutch or braces) required to walk 20 meters without resting

7.0: Unable to walk beyond 5 meters even with aid, essentially restricted to wheelchair; wheels self, transfers alone; active in wheelchair about 12 hours a day

7.5: Unable to take more than a few steps, restricted to wheelchair, may need aid to transfer; wheels self, but may require motorized chair for full day's activities

8.0: Essentially restricted to bed, chair, or wheelchair, but may be out of bed much of day; retains self care functions, generally effective use of arms

8.5: Essentially restricted to bed much of day, some effective use of arms, retains some self care functions

9.0: Helpless bed patient, can communicate and eat

9.5: Unable to communicate effectively or eat/ swallow

10.0: Death due to MS

The Expanded Disability Status Scale for evaluating MS patients.

Source: http://www.camapcanada.ca/EDSS_form_MS.pdf

Despite its advantages, there are many well-recognized problems with the EDSS. The first is that it is heavily dependent on walking and therefore may underestimate disabilities in other domains. Although patients are given a score in all of the domains of the scale, they are not all weighted equally. I have some patients who are able to walk relatively well yet have severe impairment in another domain that is not well represented in the EDSS. These include patients with visual impairment, pain, impaired cognition/psychiatric symptoms, and incontinence. Since these patients do not have significant gait impairment, their EDSS score will remain low, giving the false impression that they do not suffer from significant disability. Moreover, the same amount of disability can affect different people in different ways. One patient of mine is a fireman who had to give up his job due to mild leg weakness, while another is a lawyer who continued to work for many years though he needed a wheelchair most of the time.

A second disadvantage of the EDSS is that it is non-linear. This means that patients who have increased their EDSS score from 1 to 2 may only have a slight increase in their symptoms. In contrast, an increase from a 5 to 6 may mean the difference between being able to work or not or live independently or not. All of these patients would be deemed as having only a 1-point increase in their EDSS score, with no regard for the practical impact on their lives.

The EDSS score also needs to be interpreted over the course of a patient's illness. For example, a 60-year-old who has MS for 40 years may be doing very well if their EDSS score is 4, especially if the score has not changed in many years. In contrast, a score of 4 would be of great concern in a 25-year-old who had a lower score only a few years prior.

Finally, while the EDSS is invaluable for clinical studies, it is difficult to use it to make a treatment decision for any individual patient. I think most neurologists prefer not to use a number to make a decision about how to treat their patients. So many symptoms of MS are subjective and our patients lead such varying lives that their illness is very difficult to capture in a single score. While the EDSS is an invaluable tool for clinical trials, it cannot replace talking to and examining each patient as an individual.

31.   *Why Is MS a Difficult Disease to Study?*

There are several features of MS that make it a challenging disease to study. In other illnesses, such as many cancers, it is easy to define and measure the desired outcome—survival. If people receiving a medication survive longer than patients receiving placebo, then the medication works. Because many cancers are fatal in a relatively short period of time, trials need only last several years. By comparison, MS usually takes its toll over many decades, and most patients live 30 to 40 years after their diagnosis. How, then, do you measure the success of a medication in MS, where it can take decades for disability to develop? Clearly, it is impossible to run a clinical trial lasting 30 years.

It is also hard to define success in MS. The most commonly used outcome of success in MS trials is to measure the effect of the medication on relapse rates. Indeed, all of the MS medications decrease the number of relapses. Another universal outcome measure is the number of new brain and spinal cord lesions on MRIs. Again, the medications decrease new MRI lesions. Certainly, these outcomes are not trivial. While relapses are not usually permanently disabling, they can be psychologically devastating and expensive to treat. Moreover, it is hard to imagine that having fewer MRI lesions is not better than having more. But the long-term impact of preventing relapses and MRI lesions is surprisingly unclear.

Disability is measured in all trials as well, usually by the EDSS. This is the most important outcome in my mind, since it reflects what really matters—how patients feel and function. Though there is some variation, the medications are effective in preventing permanent disability to some degree. However, as previously discussed, disability is difficult to objectively measure. Some things, like whether a patient needs a cane to walk a certain distance, are often relatively straightforward. But other aspects of MS, such as cognition, pain, fatigue, and psychiatric symptoms, are difficult to quantify.

Lastly, getting a medication approved by the FDA is expensive and time consuming. From the time a potential medication is identified to the time it is approved by the FDA can take several decades and, by some estimates, can cost $2.6 billion.

32.   Why Should I Take a Medication if I Feel Fine?

This is one of the most common questions neurologists hear, especially early in the course of the illness. And we are certainly happy to hear it. Why would we want our patients to feel anything other than fine? However, I am always distressed when patients use this as a reason to not take a medication. After all, the point of these medications is to help ensure that people who feel fine continue to feel that way for many decades to come.

While the MS medications are effective at preventing relapses, MRI lesions, and disability, currently we are utterly unable to repair the central nervous system in any way. The cold truth is that, once a patient has a symptom for a prolonged time, it cannot be fixed. As such, neurologists want to do everything possible to prevent relapses and new symptoms before they cause permanent disability. This is why neurologists are so insistent that patients start a medication early in the disease course. Many of my older patients take multiple medications to relieve the symptoms of MS. It is my belief that had disease-modifying medications been available when they were younger, these patients would not need so many medications for their symptoms today.

For many newly diagnosed patients, the idea that an MS medication will not make them feel better when they take it (and might make them feel worse) makes no sense. Such patients are almost always otherwise healthy, active people, and in the past, they have taken only medicines that are supposed to make them feel better, such as pain relievers or antibiotics. However, the idea of taking a medicine to prevent a bad outcome is very common in medicine. No one complains that their high blood pressure or high cholesterol feels bad. Yet treatments for these conditions are among the most prescribed medications in the country, with the hope of preventing future heart attacks and strokes.

The treatments for MS are no different in that they are designed to prevent or delay *new* symptoms and disability. All of these medications work to modulate the immune system in some way. None of them repair

The Mechanism of Action of Select MS Medications: The relevant point is that they affect the immune system and do not directly affect the brain and spinal cord.

Medication	Mechanism
Gilenya	Prevents lymphocyte egress from lymph nodes by down-regulating the sphingosine 1- phosphate receptor on T-cells
Tecfidera	Activates the nuclear erythroid 2-related factor 2 transcriptional pathway
Aubagio	Inhibits dihydro-orotate dehydrogenase, a key mitochondrial enzyme in the de novo pyrimidine synthesis pathway, leading to a reduction in proliferation of lymphocytes.
Tysabri	Interferes with the $\alpha 4\beta 1$-integrin receptor molecules on the surfaces of cells, preventing lymphocyte
Lemtrada	Binds to the CD52 receptor on B and T lymphocytes
Ocrevus	Binds to CD20 positive lymphocytes

damage in the brain and spinal cord. I tend to think of MS medications as a suit of armor. If a knight was in a sword fight, their suit of armor would not heal any injuries they already received, nor would wearing that suit of armor feel good. However, it would help protect them from future injuries, though it would not guarantee their safety. Similarly, MS medications are not a cure nor do patients feel better when they take them. They are designed to prevent relapses and disability.

Whenever someone tells me they started on an MS medication but stopped it because they did not feel better, I know this person is confused about what that medication was supposed to do. It is the responsibility of the prescribing neurologist to manage the patient's expectations and properly explain the medication's purpose. Hopefully, an accurate understanding of these medications will lead to more people taking them properly.

Having said this, it may be true that not every patient needs a medication. A small number (approximately 10%) of patients have "benign" MS, where they are able to lead fully functional lives with minimal or no disability. For these patients, the medications may be unnecessary. However, there is no way at the time of diagnosis to identify which patients are destined to have benign disease, especially over the long term. For this reason, few neurologists would suggest a "wait and see" approach for a newly diagnosed patient.

Patients with clinically isolated syndrome (CIS) also present a challenge, as only time will tell if they will go on to develop MS. Patients with a single clinical demyelinating event are at risk of developing MS within years if they have two or more brain or spinal cord lesions on their MRI. Guidelines suggest that starting treatment in such patients delays the likelihood that they will experience a second event.

33. Which Medicine Should I Start Taking?

The oldest medicines in MS are the interferons and glatiramer acetate (Copaxone). The different versions of interferon are called Avonex, Betaseron, Rebif, Plegridy, and Extavia. They are very similar medications, differing primarily in their dose and the frequency they are taken. Avonex is injected once a week into the muscle, while Betaseron, Extavia, and Rebif are injected either every other day or three times per week under the skin. Plegridy is given under the skin every other week.

Copaxone is given under the skin either every day or three times per week at a higher dose. It is also available in a generic form called glatopa, which is given every day.

Drug	Betaseron Extavia	Avonex	Rebif	Plegridy	Copaxone
Year Approved	1993	1996	2002	2014	1996
Frequency	Every other Day	Weekly	3 times per week	Every 14 days	20 mg daily or 40 mg 3 times per week

The injectable medications are good for the following reasons.

THEY WORK: The effectiveness of these medicines is well-established both in clinical trials and in real-world experience. Although there may be some variability among them, they generally are effective in decreasing the annual relapse rate by about 30% to 40% and in preventing disability. There is evidence that the higher dose, higher frequency interferons, namely Betaseron, Extavia, and Rebif, are the most effective interferons. However, other studies have found that the interferons are more similar than different on a variety of efficacy measures. Similarly, the interferons and Copaxone have similar efficacy. Disability was not measured in one of the largest studies on Copaxone, the GALA trial, which studied over 1,400 patients.

THEY ARE OLD: There are 25 years of experience with the interferons and 22 years of experience with Copaxone. They have been taken by hundreds of thousands (if not millions) of people around the world. It is very unlikely that there will be any additional undiscovered harms from these medications.

THEY ARE SAFE: While these medicines are not free of side effects, serious side effects are exceedingly rare. Many patients take these medicines under the mistaken belief that they will suppress their immune system and leave them vulnerable to infections. This is not true. They are much safer than aspirin and many over-the-counter medications.

These medicines are problematic for the following reasons.

THEY ARE ALL INJECTIONS: No one likes needles. Nonetheless, all of these medications come with injecting devices that are very simple to use. Additionally, there is a large amount of support from the drug manufacturers and MS providers to help patients who have a hard time with injections. Many people have been taking these medications for over a decade. For them, the injections have become as routine as brushing their teeth. However, some people never get used to injecting themselves.

THEY HAVE SIDE EFFECTS: The interferons can cause both injection-site reactions and flu-like symptoms in a substantial number of people. Most people are able to get used to these side effects, and there are some strategies to make these medicines more tolerable. All of the interferons can be started at a low dose and gradually increased to the full dose. Many people find that taking Tylenol or Aleve before the injection limits the flu-like symptoms. Nonetheless, some people find these medicines intolerable, and for them the treatment may be worse than the disease and, of course, the treatment should never be worse than the disease.

Copaxone is only very rarely associated with systemic side effects, but patients can develop injection site reactions and occasionally cosmetically unpleasing fat breakdown at the site of the injection. Given that most people inject themselves in the thighs, buttocks, or abdomen, only intimate partners are likely to see these injection reactions.

THEY ARE NOT A CURE: While these medicines are highly effective in some patients, for many others they are simply not strong enough to prevent relapses and the accumulation of disability.

THE UPSHOT: WHO SHOULD TAKE AN INJECTABLE MEDICATION?

With the approval of more effective infusions and pills, the use of the injectable medications has decreased. However, they still have a role in the treatment of MS. Many patients have been stable on injectables for many years, and there is no reason to change their treatment. Some newly diagnosed patients wisely prefer treatments that are safe and well-established and these injectable medications are unlikely to have any surprises. If a patient starts on one of these medications and either cannot tolerate it or has continued disease activity, it is a simple matter to change their treatment.

---

34.   *What Are Monoclonal Antibodies?*

Monoclonal antibodies are large Y-shaped proteins produced by B-cells, a type of white blood cell. They are used by the immune system to identify and neutralize foreign objects, called antigens, such as bacteria and viruses.

Monoclonal antibodies are clones of a unique parent cell. Examples of monoclonal antibodies used in MS include:

- Tysabri (natilizumab)
- Lemtrada (alemtuzumab)
- Ocrevus (ocrelizumab)

35.   What Is Tysabri (natalizumab)?

Tysabri was approved by the FDA in 2004. It was the first medication that offered MS patients a treatment option beyond the injectable medications. Tysabri is given as an IV infusion every 28 days. It works by blocking a cell adhesion molecule called alpha-4-integrin, which prevents immune cells from crossing from the bloodstream into the central nervous system.

Thus far, approximately 180,000 patients have received Tysabri. Tens of thousands of people have taken it for over 6 years, and some have taken it for over a decade. Overall, there have been 618,370 patient-years of Tysabri usage (this number multiplies the number who have people who have taken a medication by how many years they have taken it.)

The efficacy of Tysabri is beyond question. In the two largest studies of Tysabri, the SENTINAL and AFFIRM trials, it showed a powerful ability to reduce disease activity in MS. In these studies, Tysabri reduced the relapse rate by 55% to 68%. Many subjects had no relapses at all. Disability progression and new MRI lesions were also significantly reduced.

Certainly, these numbers are impressive, and I don't think any neurologist would say their real-world experience deviates significantly from the results of these studies. Most of my patients on Tysabri have very boring visits (this is a good thing!), and I can remember only a couple of patients who had relapses while on Tysabri. Moreover, Tysabri is extremely well tolerated. Most patients feel nothing when they get it, and some patients even report that they feel better after taking it.

Despite its unparalleled success in treating MS, in 2005 Tysabri was temporarily removed from the market. This is because Tysabri, unlike any of the interferons or Copaxone, can cause a potentially disabling and even fatal side effect, known as progressive multifocal leukoencephalopathy (PML). PML is a viral infection of the brain caused by the JC virus. More specifically, in PML the JC virus infects oligodendrocytes, the cells in the brain that make myelin, which is the substance that is destroyed in MS. The JC virus is a very common virus, and in some studies over 70% of people have antibodies to the JC virus, indicating they were infected with it at some point in the past. It is generally a harmless virus, causing PML only in immunosuppressed individuals.

However, in patients with suppressed immune systems, the JC virus can rear its ugly head and cause PML. PML was an extremely rare diagnosis until the AIDS epidemic started in the early 1980s. Patients with PML can have widespread demyelination throughout the brain, and in patients with AIDS, the disease is often fatal. The outcome is not always so dire in patients on Tysabri, however.

As of December 2017, there have been 756 confirmed PML cases worldwide in patients on Tysabri; 25% of those patients have died.

The company that makes Tysabri continues to study its long-term effectiveness and safety in nearly 5,000 patients via the Tysabri Global Observational Program in Safety (TYGRIS) study.

36.   What Are the Risk Factors for PML in Patients on Tysabri?

Unfortunately, we can't predict for sure who will get PML. However, there are three clear risk factors that increase the chances of getting PML:

- The duration of treatment with Tysabri
- Prior treatment with immunosuppressants
- Prior exposure to the JC virus

DURATION OF TREATMENT WITH TYSABRI: The risk of PML is directly associated with the length of time someone has taken Tysabri. As of December 2017, the duration of Tysabri dosing before PML diagnosis ranged from 8 to 136 doses, while the average duration was about 49 months. It is quite safe during the first 12 to 18 months. For patients who have been on Tysabri less than 2 years, the risk of contracting PML is about 1 in 10,000. The risk seems to be the highest during the second, third, and fourth years of treatment. For people who have been on Tyrsabri for over 2 years, the risk increases to about 1 in 500 people—a substantial increase compared to patients who have been on the medicine for less than 2 years. The risk of PML does not appear to increase indefinitely, however. In fact, the risk seems to decrease after about 45 infusions. We will continue to learn as more patients stay on Tysabri for increased lengths of time.

PRIOR TREATMENT WITH IMMUNOSUPPRESSANTS: The risk of getting PML is also higher in patients who have been previously treated with immunosuppressive agents. The immunosuppressants that have been associated with

PML in patients on Tysabri include medications such as mitoxantrone, azathioprine, methotrexate, cyclophosphamide, and mycophenolate.

Although some neurologists use these medications, for the most part, they are rarely used in the treatment of MS, especially in the United States. This may be one reason that PML is more common in patients in Europe than the United States, where immunosuppressive agents are used more often. In one study, PML occurred in 3 of 2,207 patients in the United States and in 41 of 4,227 patients in Europe/Canada. Note that the interferons and Copaxone are not immunosuppressants, and prior use of these medications does not increase the risk of PML. Short courses of steroids are also not considered immunosuppressants.

EXPOSURE TO THE JC VIRUS: Patients are at greater risk if they have been exposed to the JC virus in the past. In fact, prior infection by the JC virus is basically required to develop PML. To my knowledge, there has only been a single case of a patient, a 70-year-old woman, who tested negative for the JC virus and then contracted PML soon thereafter. In another series of 278 patients who contracted PML while on Tysabri, only two were negative for the JC virus. These two patients were tested 8 and 9 months prior to the diagnosis of PML, which suggests they contracted the JC virus during this time.

Clearly, determining prior infection by the JC virus is a powerful tool for determining which patients have a negligible risk of contracting PML and which patients are more vulnerable to it. All patients considering Tysabri must be tested to determine if they have been previously infected with the JC virus and are at risk of contracting PML. Unfortunately, it is a bit more complicated than that. The JC virus is not classified as simply positive or negative. Rather, patients who test positive are given a value for how strongly they test positive. Patients with a low value (less than 0.9) have a lower risk of contracting PML. In contrast, patients who test highly positive (greater than 1.5) have a significantly elevated risk.

The range of positive values gives us significantly more information on the risk for each patient depending on how long someone has been on the medication. Assuming they have been on the medication for 5 years, if a patient's JC virus index value is below 0.9 their risk of PML is pretty low, about 1 in 2,500 people. However, it can be as high as 1 in 100 people if the index value is above 1.5. For some patients with severe MS, this 1% chance of PML might be an acceptable risk, however.

The Estimated Risk of Contracting PML Based on the JC Virus Index Value and the Length of Time on Tysabri

Length of time on Tysabri	JC index value less than 0.9	JC index value between 0.9 and 1.5	JC index value above than 1.5
1–12 months	0.01 per 1,000 people	0.1 per 1,000 people	0.2 per 1,000 people
13–24 months	0.05 per 1,000 people	0.3 per 1,000 people	0.9 per 1,000 people
25–36 months	0.2 per 1,000 people	0.8 per 1,000 people	2.6 per 1,000 people
37–48 months	0.4 per 1,000 people	2.0 per 1,000 people	6.8 per 1,000 people
49–60 months	0.5 per 1,000 people	2.4 per 1,000 people	7.9 per 1,000 people
61–72 months	0.6 per 1,000 people	3.0 per 1,000 people	10.0 per 1,000 people

Patients on Tysabri who are negative for the JC virus or those who barely test positive need to have their JC virus antibody level rechecked at least twice per year, if not more often. Though there are some conflicting data, most patients with a low or negative JC virus value continue to have a low or negative risk value. However, a small number of patients will have a large increase in their JC virus index value. It is important that these patients do not fall through the cracks and take a medication that has suddenly become much riskier for them. Moreover, there is some evidence that Tysabri itself leads to an increase in the JC virus antibody level.

Finally, there is strong evidence that giving Tysabri less frequently than every 4 weeks significantly lowers the PML risk without making the medication less effective. In one study, less frequent dosing of Tysabri was associated with a 94% lower risk for PML compared with standard dosing. Many neurologists give Tysabri every 6 or 8 weeks, in the hope that this diminishes the risk of PML.

37. How Is PML Diagnosed?

PML is diagnosed when a vulnerable patient presents with characteristic symptoms. Since PML is a brain disease, it presents with weakness, sensory changes, visual changes, language difficulties, or personality changes and cognitive deficits. As the name implies, PML is a slowly *progressive* disorder, and it usually worsens over many months.

The first step in suspected PML is to perform an MRI. Often this will reveal large areas of demyelination that look different from the lesions in MS. The lesions in PML are usually much larger and confluent than lesions in MS. Occasionally, the early changes of PML and MS lesions are indistinguishable. As such, in all cases where PML is suspected, a lumbar puncture is required to look for DNA from the JC virus in the spinal fluid. Certain laboratories are able to detect even trace amounts of this DNA. Certainly, if there is any question that a patient has PML, then Tysabri should be stopped until PML is definitively ruled-out.

Some cases of PML are detected on MRI scans before patients develop any symptoms. Most neurologists perform an MRI at least every 6 months on vulnerable patients, hoping to detect PML before any symptoms emerge. Patients who are diagnosed with PML in this early stage tend to have improved outcomes compared to patients who are diagnosed after they develop symptoms.

38.   Can PML Be Treated?

Unfortunately, there is relatively little to do to directly treat PML, and there are no clinical trials to guide treatment. Many neurologists feel the first step is to remove Tysabri from a patient's bloodstream, especially if they recently received an infusion. This is done via a procedure called plasmapheresis, which often requires that patients be admitted to the hospital. This effectively removes Tysabri from the body allowing for the immune system to recover. It is usually done for several days in a row.

There are no FDA-approved medications that target the JC virus directly. There have been reports of successful treatment in a small number of patients with antiviral drugs, antimalarial drugs, and chemotherapeutic agents. One encouraging sign is that, unlike in patients with AIDS, a fair number of Tysabri patients with PML have been able to survive the infection with minimal disability. This seems to be the case for more recent cases of PML now that neurologists are on high alert against the infection and stop Tysabri as soon as PML is suspected. However, as previously mentioned, PML has been fatal in nearly 25% of patients thus far, and many survivors are left with significant disability.

Clearly, PML is a serious disease. Hopefully, we can continue to make more accurate predictions about which patients are at the highest risk of contracting PML and for whom Tysabri should not even be considered.

Additionally, we hope to have effective treatments for the unfortunate patients who contract this disease.

THE UPSHOT: WHO SHOULD TAKE TYSABRI?

For patients who test negative for the JC virus, the risk of contracting PML is very low (less than 1 in 10,000). I do not hesitate to suggest Tysabri for JC virus negative patients if there is any indication that less powerful medications cannot control their disease.

In contrast, patients who test positive for the JC virus antibody need to have highly active disease to justify the use of Tysabri. There is no agreement on what is meant by "active disease," however. It is up to neurologists and patients to try to strike the right balance between the risk posed by the medicine and the risk posed by the disease. Just like there is no "right" amount of money everyone should save for retirement, there is no "right" answer about when the risks of Tysabri outweigh the benefits. Some patients are terrified of their MS. Others are more fearful of the medication.

Patients who experience an infusion-reaction or have disease activity when receiving Tysabri may have developed neutralizing antibodies that lessen the efficacy of the medication. Neurologists should check for such antibodies in appropriate patients.

39.   What Is Lemtrada (alemtuzumab)?

Lemtrada is a monoclonal antibody that binds to certain immune cells. It is also approved for the treatment of B-cell chronic lymphocytic leukemia. It gained FDA approval for MS in 2014. It is given by IV infusion for 5 days initially and then for 3 days 1 year later. This means it is only given eight times over 3 years. The large studies of Lemtrada are known as the CARE-MS I and II trials. In these trials, Lemtrada was compared to Rebif, an older, standard treatment for MS. In both trials, Lemtrada reduced relapses by 49% to 55%. Over half of patients on Lemtrada had no relapses after 2 years, and the average EDSS score for patients treated with Lemtrada *decreased*, indicating an improvement in physical disability. Multiple aspects of MRI-detected disease activity also showed benefit in patients who received Lemtrada.

Subjects in the CARE-MS I and II trials were followed for 5 years after the official end of the trials, and Lemtrada continued to show impressive efficacy. Even though nearly 60% of subjects did not receive Lemtrada after the trials ended, 75% of them did not show any clinical worsening and some continued to show improvement in their disability. Its performance in these trials is even more impressive given that it was compared to an effective medication for MS, not an inert placebo.

Unfortunately, Lemtrada has some potentially significant side effects. The most serious complication is a platelet disorder called immune thrombocytopenic purpura (ITP), which occurs in about 1% of patients. This included a study subject who died from uncontrolled bleeding. After the first cases of ITP occurred, the drug company implemented a safety monitoring program. All subsequent cases of ITP were detected early through a monitoring program and successfully managed with conventional therapies. Infections in those treated with Lemtrada were mild to moderate. Additionally, about 16% of patients developed autoimmune thyroid-related problems. Other common adverse events, such as headache, rash, fever, flushing, hives, and chills, were related to infusion of Lemtrada.

THE UPSHOT: WHO SHOULD TAKE LEMTRADA?

Lemtrada is a powerful medicine and a great option for some patients. It is dosed very infrequently and its onset of action is very rapid. It is most appropriate as a second- or third-line treatment in patients with aggressive disease who are not good candidates for Tysabri. It can be used as a first-line treatment for a small number of patients with very aggressive disease.

The main downside is that patients will have to get monthly blood draws, though often these can be arranged at their house or job. This means that Lemtrada can only be given to very reliable patients. Patients who miss appointments and blood draws will not be good candidates for this medicine. Patients also need to carefully monitor themselves for any rash that might indicate ITP and notify their doctor immediately if any rash emerges. The rash is usually minute, red/purple spots called petechiae. Other warning signs of ITP include easy or excessive bruising, blood in the urine or stool, bleeding from the gums or nose, and an unusually heavy menstrual flow.

40.   What Is Ocrevus (ocrelizumab)?

Ocrevus was approved by the FDA in 2017. It is virtually identical to an older medication called Rituxan (rituximab), which has also shown efficacy in MS. Ocrevus initially is given twice as an infusion 2 weeks apart and then as a single infusion every 6 months. As of July 2018, it has been taken by about 50,000 patients. The main trials in relapsing-remitting MS (RRMS) were the OPERA I and II trials. The OPERA I and II trials were two identical trials where Ocrevus was compared to Rebif, which is considered one of the more powerful interferons. They found that Ocrevus reduced the relapse rate by 46% to 47% percent compared to Rebif. Ocrevus also reduced new MRI lesions and disability compared to Rebif. The percentage of patients with No Evidence of Disease Activity (NEDA) was also improved.

Importantly, Ocrevus was the first medicine to show efficacy in primary progressive MS (PPMS). This was shown in the ORATORIO trial, which compared Ocrevus to placebo. In this trial there was a 24% reduction in this risk of 12- and 24-week confirmed disability progression. Patients who received Ocrevus also had fewer new MRI lesions and less decline in their ability to walk 25 feet.

Clearly, Ocrevus is a very effective medication in RRMS. It is also the first medication approved for PPMS. Because it is given every 6 months, it is very convenient as well. It is generally very well tolerated and most people feel nothing when they receive the infusion.

There was a small hint of increased cancers in patients taking Ocrevus. In the OPERA studies, there were 2 cancers out of 826 subjects who received Rebif and 6 cancers out of 825 subjects who received Ocrevus. None of these were fatal. In the ORATORIO study, there were 2 cancers out of 239 patients who received placebo and 11 cancers out of 486 subjects who received Ocrevus. One patient who received Ocrevus died of pancreatic cancer. The cancers were not in a particular organ and there were several

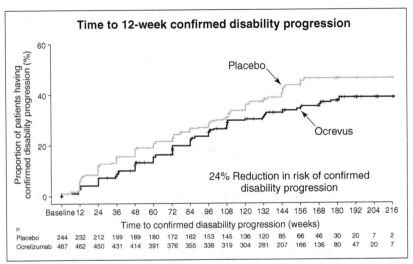

The proportion of patients who had disability progression while on placebo (top line) and Ocrevus (bottom line). As you can see, people who received Ocrevus had less disability progression.

basal cell carcinomas, an easily treatable skin cancer. Overall, the cancer rate was *not* higher with Ocrevus than is expected in the general population. Also, Ocrevus is virtually identical to Rituxan, a medication that has been used for many years and which is not known to cause cancer on its own.

Thus far, there is no signal that patients who take Ocrevus are at a higher risk for serious infections. Ocrevus was being investigated as a treatment for rheumatoid arthritis, but the company stopped the studies due to serious and sometimes fatal infections. However, rheumatoid arthritis is a different disease than MS, and the infections occurred when Ocrevus was combined with other immunosuppressant medications. Thus far, there have been no cases of PML in patients on Ocrevus alone, though there have been two cases in patients who had previously taken Gilenya and Tysabri. Most likely, the use of these medications was responsible for the PML.

THE UPSHOT: WHO SHOULD TAKE OCREVUS?

In a short amount of time, Ocrevus has become one of the most widely used medications in MS. It appears to have everything going for it. It is certainly effective. It is also very tolerable and convenient for patients to take. At this time, it also appears safe. As such, it is appropriate for nearly all patients with RRMS, and it is the only option for patients with PPMS. It is most effective in PPMS patients who are still walking. It is not clear that it helps patients who can no longer walk. Clearly, the potential for increased cancers and infections needs to be closely monitored now that the medicine is being widely used in the real world.

41. What About the Oral Medications?

The three oral medications in MS are Gilenya, Aubagio, and Tecfidera. These medications have ushered in a new era of treatment for patients with MS. While they all have different risk and benefit profiles, overall I think they have a very favorable combination of safety, efficacy, and tolerability. These medications are widely used in many MS patients. Unfortunately,

The Oral Medications

Drug	Gilenya	Aubagio	Tecfidera
Year Approved	2010	2012	2013
Frequency	Daily	Daily	Twice daily
Efficacy	Lowers relapses by about 50%	Lowers relapses by about 33%	Lowers relapses by about 50%

they are not a cure, and some patients continue to have active disease while on these medications.

42. What Is Gilenya (fingolimod)?

In 2010, the FDA approved the first oral medication for RRMS, Gilenya. In 2018, this became the first medication approved for children over the age of 10 years. It is taken once daily. It is derived from a fungus and blocks the sphingosine-1-phosphate receptor, which is found mainly on lymph nodes. Blocking this receptor traps certain immune cells, known as lymphocytes, in lymph nodes. This prevents them from reaching the central nervous system, where they cause inflammation, relapses, and disability. It is hoped that Gilenya only minimally interferes with the overall health of the immune function because the lymphocytes are still active within the lymphatic system.

The main studies of Gilenya were the FREEDOMS, FREEDOMS II, and the TRANSFORMS trials. In these studies, Gilenya reduced relapses by 48% to 54% and also reduced new MRI lesions. Subjects on Gilenya had a higher incidence of herpes zoster, lower respiratory tract infections, influenza, macular edema, and basal cell carcinomas. There were two fatal infections, one from disseminated primary varicella zoster (the virus that causes chickenpox) and one from herpes simplex encephalitis. These patients were taking higher doses of Gilenya than was approved by the FDA.

The participants in these three studies continue to be monitored to evaluate Gilenya's long-term efficacy and safety. As with any medication, the news on Gilenya can be divided into the good and the bad. Let's talk about the good news first.

IT IS A PILL: Many patients have a fear of needles that makes them unable to take the injectable medications. The introduction of an oral medication meant that, for the first time, these patients could treat their MS without a needle. Other patients aren't afraid of needles but simply cannot tolerate the side effects from the injectable medications. Patients on Gilenya are spared the flu-like symptoms that often occur with the interferons or the injection-site reactions that can occur with any injectable medication.

IT WORKS: In the FREEDOMS trials, Gilenya was found to be superior to placebo and Avoenx (one of the older interferons) in preventing relapses, preventing disability progression, and in new lesions on the MRI. Although no direct comparisons have ever been done in a clinical trial, some studies have shown Gilenya is as effective as Tysabri. Other studies, however, have concluded that Gilenya is not as effective as Tysabri.

IT IS TOLERABLE: In the FREEDOMS trial, about 20% of the patients receiving Gilenya 0.5 mg stopped taking the medication before the trial was over, while nearly 30% of patients taking placebo did so. In the TRANFORMS study, the discontinuation rates between patients taking the Gilenya 0.5 mg dose and Avonex were equal. In both trials, there were slightly higher rates of discontinuation of the higher dose of Gilenya, but, again, this was not the dose approved by the FDA. In the real world, I have found that very few patients have tolerability issues with Gilenya.

43. What Are the Downsides to Gileyna?

IT IS NEW, BUT NOT THAT NEW: In contrast to the injectable medications, Gilenya is a relative "baby" with unknown long-term side effects. Still, it is not *that* new anymore. It was approved in 2010, and as of this writing, it has been taken by over 255,000 patients. So patients who wish to start Gilenya now should know that there is experience with it, but not as much as with the interferons and Copaxone.

IT HAS SOME SIDE EFFECTS: The very first dose of Gilenya can slow patients' heart rates. For this reason, patients have to be monitored for the first 6 hours after taking the medication. There have been a handful of cases of bradycardia (slow heart rate) in patients taking their first dose. This suggests that the medication should probably not be used in patients with cardiac disease. However, very few newly diagnosed patients have any heart condition. Moreover, the first-dose monitoring can now be done at home for most patients. Fortunately, the slow heart rate during the first dose of Gilenya has not turned out to be a significant concern.

Gilenya can also cause an eye condition called macular edema. This is generally a benign condition that is reversible when Gilenya is stopped, and occurs in less than 1% of people. Still, patients have to see an eye doctor prior to starting Gilenya and periodically thereafter to monitor for this condition. A common problem with Gilenya is complications of the varicella zoster virus. This is the virus that causes chickenpox in kids and shingles in adults. Shingles can be a serious disease, causing a painful rash at minimum. At times it can lead to strokes or directly affect the brain or spinal cord. Everyone should be checked for exposure to chickenpox prior to starting Gilenya. Adults over the age of 50 should consider getting the shingles vaccine, though there is some concern that live vaccines are unsafe in MS. Additionally, in the clinical trials of Gilenya, there were several deaths due to infections, including one death from varicella zoster virus. These deaths occurred at a higher dose of Gilenya than was approved by the FDA, however.

Now that Gilenya has been in the real world for some time, other infections have begun to emerge. As of February 2018, there have been 21 cases of PML. All but one of these occurred in patients older than 50 years old. As of February 2018, there have also been have been 35 reported cases of cryptococcal meningitis. This is a fungal infection most commonly seen in patients with AIDS. Of these 35 cases, 9 people died.

There is some evidence that taking Gilenya every other day is as effective as taking it every day. This is a reasonable strategy in patients who develop a low white blood cell count, which is very common with Gilenya. It is hoped that the risk of these infections can be minimized by taking Gilenya less often.

There is a concern that Gilenya may predispose patients to skin cancers, such as basal cell carcinoma and melanoma. Unfortunately, a large trial of Gilenya in patients with primary-progressive MS showed no benefit.

GILENYA DOES NOT SEEM SAFE IN PREGNANCY: There have been 5 cases of abnormal fetal development among 66 pregnancies in women taking Gilenya. In all 5 cases, fetal exposure took place in the first trimester. Therefore, all sexually active women should practice safe sex while on Gilenya.

THE UPSHOT: WHO SHOULD TAKE GILENYA?

Gilenya is most appropriate for young, otherwise healthy patients who either cannot tolerate the injections or have MS that is poorly controlled by other medications. It is also completely reasonable to start newly diagnosed patients on Gilenya. Most patients on Gilenya are very happy with the medication thus far. Because of the first-dose cardiac monitoring and need for an eye exam, it is a bit of a pain to start compared other medications. Gilenya comes with rare, but real risks. To my knowledge, there have been serious infections in about 60 patients thus far. Given that over 225,000 people have taken Gilenya, the risk of a serious infection is about 1 in 4,000 patients. While this risk is very low, it is not zero. Each patient must decide for themselves if they find this an acceptable risk or not. Patients who are negative for the JC virus and younger than 50 years are at lower risk, at least for PML.

Several medications that are similar to Gilenya (ozanimod, ponesimod, and siponimod) may be approved soon. They will be easier to start as there is no need for cardiac monitoring or eye exams. Siponimod has also shown some efficacy in SPMS.

44.   What Is Aubagio (teriflunomide)?

Aubagio was the second pill for MS, approved by the FDA in 2012. Aubagio is the active metabolite of Arava (leflunimode), a medication that was approved by the FDA in 1998 for rheumatoid arthritis. In this sense, it is not really new. Aubagio works by inhibiting an enzyme in the synthesis of DNA. This disrupts the function of both T- and B-lymphocytes, each of which has been implicated in inflammation and injury in MS. It only affects the more rapidly dividing cells of the immune system and so has a limited effect on the immune system as a whole. It is taken once daily, and there are two doses, 7 mg and 14 mg. The main studies of Aubagio are the TOWER and TEMSO trials. In these trials, Aubagio reduced relapses by 22% to 36%. Subjects taking Aubagio experienced more headache, nausea, diarrhea, hair thinning, and low levels of white blood cells. In a study called the TOPIC trial, subjects with clinically isolated syndrome (CIS) who were at high risk for developing MS found that Aubagio reduced the risk of people developing MS compared to placebo.

Aubagio has also been studied in combination with the injectable medications. A small trial combining Aubagio and an interferon showed that this combination led to an improvement in several MRI measures and appeared to reduce the relapse rate compared with Aubagio alone. Another small study found that Aubagio combined with Copaxone reduced MRI lesions compared to Copaxone alone.

Numerous subjects have taken Aubagio as part of these studies, some for nearly 10 years. Thus far, it appears to be a very safe and generally well-tolerated medication. Though patients need to have liver function tests monitored once a month for the first 6 months of treatment, I am unaware of any serious side effects that are directly related to Aubagio.

All sexually active women need to practice birth control while on Aubagio and have a negative pregnancy test prior to starting it. It is considered category X in pregnancy. This sounds scary, but it simply means that there is no evidence of harm or safety in pregnant women. However, there is evidence of harm in animal studies, though these are usually done at much higher doses than that taken by people. Thus far, 83 pregnancies have been recorded in women while taking Aubagio, without evidence of harm. However, as birth defects are not rare in even the best of circumstances, I worry that it will be held responsible, rightly or not, for any birth defect. Therefore, any woman who becomes pregnant or intends to become pregnant while on Aubagio, needs to take a second medication to purge Aubagio out of their system.

THE UPSHOT: WHO SHOULD TAKE AUBAGIO?

Aubagio is a moderately effective medication that is most appropriate for patients with relatively mild disease. Though Aubagio is not the most powerful medication, it is the only one of the oral medications not to have any cases of PML thus far. It is appropriate for patients who prioritize safety over efficacy. Though patients need to have their liver checked every month for 6 months, patients almost never have to stop taking Aubagio due to liver damage. Many patients are also fearful when they learn that hair thinning is a possible side effect. However, this occurs in a very small number of patients and usually only at the start of treatment. Even then, it is not permanent. All women taking Aubagio should practice safe sex, and need to take another medication to remove Aubagio from their system if they become pregnant.

45. What Is Tecfidera (dimethyl fumarate)?

Tecfidera was approved by the FDA in 2013. It is a pill that is taken twice daily. Tecfidera is very similar to another medication called Fumaderm, which has been used since 1994 to treat psoriasis, primarily in Germany. As such, it is not really that new a medication. There were no deaths or serious adverse events related to Tecfidera. There was no increase in the overall number of infections, serious infections, or cancers.

Shortly after Tecfidera's approval by the FDA, it emerged that there were several cases of PML in patients taking Fumaderm. However, in some of these cases, the patients were on other drugs that suppress the immune system and lead to PML. These patients also had very low white blood cell counts for a prolonged period of time. In 2014, the first MS patient taking Tecfidera was diagnosed with PML. This patient, like those on Fumaderm, had been taking Tecfidera for nearly 5 years and had a very low white blood cell count.

Thus far, there have been five cases of PML in MS patients taking Tecfidera. Considering that over 250,000 people have taken it, the risk of PML is very low. Still, it is something that needs to be considered. As a persistently low white blood cell count may be a risk for PML, stopping Tecfidera might be indicated in such patients. There have also been 14 reported cases of liver injury in patients taking Tecfidera, though none went into liver failure and all cases recovered once the drug was stopped.

Unfortunately, the use of Tecfidera has been limited by problems with its tolerability. The medication is given twice daily, and for some patients, having to remember to take a pill this often is a significant burden (though missing a dose here or there is not a big deal). The most common side effects of Tecfidera are flushing and gastrointestinal upset. About 40% of patients experience flushing. However, this abates over several months in most patients and only 3% of patients in clinical trials stopped Tecfidera for this reason. Gastrointestinal tract irritation (abdominal pain, diarrhea nausea, and vomiting) is also a common side effect. It similarly tends to abate after 1 month of treatment in most patients, and only 4% of subjects in clinical trials discontinued Tecfidera for this reason.

There are several tips to minimize the side effects:

- Take Tecfidera with food or with 2 tablespoons of peanut butter (if no nut allergies)

- If flushing occurs, take 81mg *non-enteric coated* aspirin 30 minutes before taking Tecfidera

- Take Pepto-Bismol/Kaopectate for nausea/diarrhea as needed

- Stop any medication used for bowel regulation while taking Tecfidera

The use of an allergy medication called Singulair may also be helpful. Additionally, by starting out at a small dose and gradually escalating to the full dose, both the flushing and gastrointestinal upset can be minimized. A Tecfidera dosing schedule is shown below:

- Week 1 and 2 (14 days): Take 120 mg (green and white capsule) *ONCE* a day with a meal consisting of healthy fats.

- Week 3 and 4 (14 days): Take 240 mg (green capsule) *ONCE* a day with a meal consisting of healthy fats.

- Week 5 (maintenance dose): Take 240 mg capsule *TWO TIMES* daily (minimum of 8 hours between doses)

Despite these techniques, the side effects can make it difficult for some patients to tolerate Tecfidera. Indeed, one study found that after 2 years, over 50% of patients stopped taking Tecfidera because of these side effects or lack of efficacy.

THE UPSHOT: WHO SHOULD TAKE TECFIDERA?

Tecfidera is an effective and safe medication for preventing relapses and slowing disease progression in MS. It is a pill and is more effective than Copaxone, one of the oldest treatments in MS. It is appropriate for almost all patients with RRMS. Though some patients are unable to tolerate its side effects, few serious safety concerns have emerged. PML has occurred in about 1 in 50,000 patients this far, a risk that most people find acceptable.

46. PML Summary

As of this writing, there have been five PML cases with Tecfidera out of about 250,000 patients, 19 PML cases with Gilenya out of about 255,000 patients, and 756 PML cases in Tysabri out of about 180,000 patients. The risk with these medications is presented in the table below.

The PML Risk With Various MS Treatments

Drug	Tysabri	Gilenya	Tecfidera
PML Risk	756 cases out of 180,000 patients	21 cases out of 255,000 patients	5 cases out of 250,000 patients

47. What Is Novantrone (mitoxantrone)?

Novantrone is a chemotherapeutic agent that was approved in 2000. It is used for both aggressive SPMS and RRMS. It inserts itself into DNA strands affecting the proliferation of cells of the immune system. It is the only medication approved for SPMS and it is given as IV infusion every 3 months. Though it is effective in slowing the course of SPMS, its use is limited by the potential for infertility, leukemia, and injury to heart muscles. Due to these side effects, there is a maximum lifetime dose patients may receive. Regular cardiac monitoring is required for patients who have received Novantrone. Other side effects include nausea/vomiting, hair loss, loss of menstruation, suppression of the bone marrow, and urinary and respiratory tract infections. Most MS specialists do not use this medication any more, though it still has a role in patients with rapidly-advancing SPMS.

48. How Do I Know if My Medication Is Working?

There are three reasons to change a medication in someone with MS:

- They cannot tolerate the medication.
- The medication is felt to be too unsafe.
- The medication is not controlling their MS.

One of the hardest questions patients ask is whether or not their medication is working. Some patients have had many relapses before they decide to start a medication. If their relapses greatly diminish after this, it is fair to assume that the medication is working for them. However, for newly diagnosed patients, it can be very difficult to tell if their treatment is working. The medications are designed to prevent bad things from happening, and they do this with varying levels of effectiveness. However, this makes it impossible to know what negative events, if any, a medication may have prevented in any given patient. This is not unique to MS, of course. As stated previously, the treatment of conditions such as high blood pressure and high cholesterol is meant primarily to prevent cardiovascular disease.

One area of disagreement among neurologists is that there is no consensus on what is meant by "treatment failure." If a patient relapses every 3 years, does that mean the medication is working or not? Perhaps without the medication, the patient would have had many more relapses. It is impossible to say. Most neurologists would switch a patient's medication to a more powerful treatment if they had a relapse every 3 years. However, other neurologists might disagree and say this is not a reason to expose a patient to a more aggressive and potentially riskier treatment. Similarly, there is also no universal agreement about what to do with patients who feel well but have new MRI lesions. However, recent guidelines from the American Academy of Neurology suggest considering changing medications in patients who have taken a medication for 1 year and experienced either a single new relapse, two new MRI lesions, or increased disability.

Some patients tell me, correctly, that their MS has worsened after taking a medication. Once again, is this due to the ineffectiveness of the medication or due to disease progression? Another analogy is in order. Let's imagine there was a pill that cut the aging process in half. This would be amazing! We all would take it. But after taking it for 40 years, everyone would feel 20 years older. So someone who used this miracle pill would rightly say they continued to age while taking it. The same may be true for MS patients. While their MS has worsened on a medication, it likely would have worsened more rapidly had they never taken it.

Clearly, the medication trials demonstrate that patients who take medications do better than those who don't. However, the only way to know for sure if a medication is working in any individual would be to clone them and have them lead two lives, one where they take the medicine and one where they do not. Often, there is no way to be certain whether a medication is working in any individual. However, even in patients who continue to have relapses and increased disability while on a medication, I believe that most of them would be even worse off without it, but I cannot say that for sure.

Ultimately, whether a medication is "working" or not depends on the individual patient. It is uncertainties such as this, however, that make medicine, especially neurology, an art as much as a science.

Lastly, there is an understandable and natural tendency for many people to hold a medication responsible for any problem they might experience after they start it. It is important not to blame everything bad that happens after starting a medication on that medication. In the clinical trials, patients who take a harmless placebo sometimes develop serious, even fatal diseases (this is called the nocebo effect). This proves that bad things can happen to people independent of the medication they take.

Side effects listed on the medication label are often not helpful either. These lists are made by drug companies to protect themselves from lawsuits, not to inform doctors and patients. According to one study, the average drug label lists 70 possible side effects and some list over 500. Some common symptoms, like nausea, are listed as a side effect of almost every medication. Several patients of mine have discarded perfectly good treatments, I believe, as they blamed them for problems that are almost certainly unrelated to the medication. I feel this is a mistake.

49. What Is Dangerous for Patients with MS?

In judging the risks of MS medications, I always like to keep other risks in perspective. We are often not afraid of dangerous things, and we are often terrified by things that are quite safe. This is just human nature. Certainly, fires, falls, and suicide pose a much greater risk than most MS medications. Many patients engage in relatively dangerous activities, such as riding in a car or swimming, without a second thought, yet they are terrified of MS medications, even though they are much safer. Even in the most high-risk patients, the risk of contracting PML while on Tysabri is about the same as dying in a car crash. Following is a list of what actually killed Americans in 2016. I find it useful to refer to this chart when thinking about the dangers of MS medications.

50. Will I Have to Take This Medication for the Rest of My Life?

For most patients, the idea of starting an MS treatment is daunting for several reasons. One reason is the fear that they will have to take a medication for many decades. While young, newly diagnosed patients can expect to be on a medication for many years, I do not believe that all patients will be on one for the rest of their lives. As described, the medications are

Lifetime Odds of Death in the United States (2016)	
Cause of Death	Odds of Dying
Heart Disease	1 in 6
Cancer	1 in 7
Chronic Lower Respiratory Disease	1 in 27
Suicide	1 in 91
Motor Vehicle Crash	1 in 102
Opioid Pain Killer Overdoses	1 in 109
Fall	1 in 119
Gun Assault	1 in 285
Pedestrian Incident	1 in 561
Motorcyclist	1 in 846
Drowning	1 in 1,086
Fire or Smoke	1 in 1,506
Choking on Food	1 in 3,138
Bicyclist	1 in 4,050
Accidental Gun Discharge	1 in 8,305
Sunstroke	1 in 8,976
Electrocution, Radiation, Extreme Temperatures and Pressure	1 in 14,630
Sharp Objects	1 in 27,407
Hornet, Wasp and Bee Stings	1 in 54,093
Hot Surfaces and Substances	1 in 56,316
Cataclysmic Storm	1 in 62,288
Lightning	1 in 114,195
Dog Attack	1 in 132,614
Railway Passenger	1 in 178,741
Passenger on an Airplane	1 in 205,552

The odds of dying according to the National Safety Counsel (2016).

primarily intended to prevent relapses, which tend to naturally decrease as patients age.

The data thus far on patients who stopped their medications are mixed. In one study, patients with stable MS over the age of 40 found that 40% of them had some disease activity return after they stopped taking medication; 42% of these patients restarted the medication or started a new one. However, another study tracked patients older than 60 who stopped their medication. Only 1% of these patients experienced a relapse, and only 11% ended up restarting a medication.

Currently, a trial is ongoing to determine which patients, if any, can safely stop their MS medication. It is enrolling patients older than 55 who have been on a medication for several years without any clinical change or new MRI lesions. Half of these patients will continue their medication, while the other half will stop it. The results will help determine if older, stable patients can safely stop their medications. Patients with CIS may also consider stopping if they have not had a relapse or new MRI lesion for 2 years. All patients who stop medications should check in with their neurologist at least once per year and get repeat MRIs on a regular basis to make sure there are no new lesions.

51. Can Medications Be Combined?

It makes intuitive sense that combining MS medications would lead to improved outcomes. As the medications work by different mechanisms, this might allow MS to be attacked from two different angles. At present, however, there is little evidence that combining MS treatments leads to greater efficacy or safety. The largest study to investigate combining MS therapies found there was no benefit to combining an interferon and Copaxone. It's possible that oral medications might be combined with the older, injectable medications. Aubagio combined with Copaxone was safe, well-tolerated, and reduced some MRI markers of disease activity. Another trial studied whether Aubagio combined with interferon beta was safe and effective, though the results have not been released yet. Another study is investigating if ponesimod, a medication similar to Gilenya, can be safely and effectively combined with Tecfidera.

52. What About Stem Cells?

Stem cells are unquestionably one of the hottest topics in MS. A group from Canada made headlines by treating 24 patients with stem cells. All but one patient were relapse-free for as long as 13 years. Another study in 2018 also garnered significant attention. It compared 110 patients who either received stem cells or a standard MS treatment. After 1 year, there was only one relapse in the 55 patients who received stem cells, while the 55 subjects who took medications had 39 relapses. Patients who received the stem cells also had improved disability scores. The lead neurologist behind this study, Dr. Richard Burt, said, "The data are stunningly in favor of transplant against the best available drugs—the neurological community has been skeptical about this treatment, but these results will change that."

When people hear about stem cells, they often ascribe to them almost magical properties, namely the ability to repair injuries to the brain and spine. Unfortunately, the science is not there yet, despite sensational headlines such as "Stem-Cell Treatment Beats Medicine in Severe Multiple Sclerosis." Despite what many people think, stem cells do not go into the brain and spinal cord to repair injured nervous tissues. What the sensational headlines omit is that patients receive "intense immunosuppression" before receiving the stem cells. It is this immunosuppression that controls MS. Some stem cell protocols use Lemtrada (alemtuzumab), which is already approved for MS, while others use large doses of chemotherapy. Stem cells are then given *after* the chemotherapy to "reboot" the immune system.

While this treatment has shown great results, its potential for toxicity means that it should be reserved only for the small number of patients with the most aggressive disease who continue to have multiple relapses and substantial disability progression while on safer treatments. In the Canadian study, for example, 1 of the 24 patients died of liver failure and overwhelming infections attributed to the chemotherapy regimen. Deaths have occurred in other MS patients who received stem cells, and one prominent researcher received a warning letter from the FDA for not properly reporting these deaths and other serious side effects.

Other groups are investigating stem cell therapies in different ways. These treatments involve injecting stem cells into the spinal column or intravenously. It is too early to comment on the safety and efficacy of these treatments. Right now, they are investigational and I do not think patients should take the risk and expense of these treatments unless they are involved in a clinical trial. Several of my patients have traveled to other countries and paid thousands of dollars for unproven and potentially dangerous treatments. I understand that people are desperate to feel better, but I believe they were taken advantage of by unethical doctors.

When stem cells are given intravenously or directly into the spinal fluid, there is no guarantee that the cells will get to the right place in the brain, there is no guarantee that they will remyelinate axons, and there is no guarantee that they will not overgrow. Indeed, a memorable headline about the dangers of stem cells read "Woman Grows Nose Tumor in Spine After Stem Cell Experiment." *The New York Times* also reported the case of an unfortunate stroke victim who grew a tumor on his spine and became paralyzed after getting stem cells injected in his spinal column. This man had some wise advice, saying, "Don't trust anecdotes." His sister-in-law had a different reply: "If something sounds too good to be true, it is."

So, while there is great potential with stem cells, there is a need to move cautiously.

53.   What About Treating Pediatric MS?

Relapses in pediatric MS are treated with steroids the same as for adults. Plasmapheresis can be used in severe relapses. The disease-modifying therapies that reduce relapses in adults are also extremely effective in children under 18 years of age, including much younger children. It's even possible that the medications are more effective in children. The only medication that is FDA approved for children over 10 years of age, however, is Gilenya. It gained this approval in May 2018.

In addition to taking medications, it's important for children with MS to exercise regularly, to continue to participate in sports and social activities, to maintain active social interactions with friends, and to eat a healthy, balanced diet. One study showed that those children whose calories came from fruits, vegetables, and polyunsaturated fats were less likely to experience a relapse compared to those who ate fewer fruits and vegetables and more saturated fats.

Sometimes young people with MS need some help in coping with having a medical condition. More often, children handle the diagnosis well. On the other hand, it can be very challenging for some parents to have a child with a serious medical condition. It is reassuring that children with MS generally do so well. Further, support groups for parents can alleviate many concerns and talking with the neurologist can be helpful. Lastly, children with MS or their guardian should request extra time when taking tests or request additional help in school if they need it.

54.   Why Is Progress in MS So Difficult?

Although it may seem that progress in MS is slow, the treatment landscape has changed dramatically in the past few years. Prior to 1993, there were exactly zero drugs approved to treat MS. Since 2010, three oral medications have been approved as have two powerful infusions and a medication to improve walking in patients with MS. Several other disease-modifying medications (ofatumumab, ozanimod, ponesimod, laquinimod, siponimod, and cladribine) may be approved in the near future. Stem cells have shown amazing efficacy in a small number of patients and may become a more common treatment in the future as well. Improving symptomatic treatments is also an active area of investigation. A lab test called neurofilament light chain is being investigated as a means of predicting disease activity and severity.

Despite these successes and potential new developments, progress is not as fast as we want. There is still no cure. There are several reasons why it is difficult to conduct clinical trials of new MS medications. Finding potential treatments takes many years of scientific research. Once a potential new drug is identified, it takes many more years to properly study it. Drug trials must enroll hundreds of volunteer subjects around the world and multiple studies must be done. It costs several billion dollars before a drug is approved by the FDA. For every successful drug, there are many costly failures.

It can also be very difficult to get patients to enroll in studies of MS medications. In the days before treatments were available, enrolling patients in clinical trials was easy. Now, few patients want to be "guinea pigs." This is a problem, as our knowledge of MS (and other diseases) will only advance if patients are willing to enroll in studies. Patients should be strongly encouraged to participate in research as long as they feel it is safe and appropriate for them. Patients who participate in research are doing something heroic that will benefit people in the future. The Multiple Sclerosis Society has a list of ongoing clinical trials on its website.

Scientists and drug companies face many significant hurdles in studying medications for MS. However, there is a lot of research going on to try to slow down the disease course, improve symptoms, and repair damage to the nervous system. Several new medications and treatments are being studied. These include truly imaginative ways of shutting down the immune system, such as purposely infecting patients with parasitic worms to dampen down the immune system. Repairing damaged myelin and axons is truly the holy grail of MS, though the one medication studied for this purpose failed.

Patients today have many more options to treat MS than in the past. I have no doubt that in the future many more options will emerge. The Multiple Sclerosis Society webpage is a good place to check for the latest research and developments. I hope this section provided an explanation as to why development of new MS treatments is often slower than anyone would like.

55. Should I Take Any Supplements?

A large number of supplements and vitamins have been proposed to treat MS. These include:

- Omega-3 fatty acids
- Linoleic acid
- Cod liver oil
- Probiotics
- Vitamin B12
- Selenium
- Ginkgo biloba extracts
- Coenzyme Q10
- Vitamin D

By some estimates, over half of MS patients take some supplements. However, a large review in 2012 from the Cochrane Database of Systematic Reviews found that proper studies on vitamins and supplements simply have not been done in MS. When it came to evaluating the adequacy of studies of vitamins and supplements, the authors reported that "No studies on vitamins and antioxidant supplements were found that met our criteria." In other words, there really have not been any large, well-controlled studies of vitamins and supplements in MS. According to the review paper, "Evidence bearing on the possible benefits and risks of vitamin supplementation and antioxidant supplements in MS is lacking. More research is required to assess the effectiveness of diet interventions in MS."

Though many patients take numerous supplements and vitamins, for most of them, there is no evidence they do any good. Fortunately, vitamin deficiencies are vanishingly rare in the United States. This is why diseases like scurvy, rickets, and pellagra are largely relegated to the history books. Based on the available evidence, I do not believe supplements offer any particular benefit to patients with MS, though I am optimistic that further studies will support a role for vitamin D.

I am also concerned that untested supplements and vitamins may have unforeseen side effects. Many patients feel these products are safe because they feel they are taking something "natural." Most likely, such supplements will be excreted harmlessly in the urine. However, it is a mistake to say that just because something is "natural" it must be harmless and without side effects. Few people would eat random berries and mushrooms they found in a forest simply because these are "natural."

Moreover, there is nothing natural about taking extremely large doses of vitamins and supplements. Too much of *anything* can be dangerous. There is a rule in medicine that "the dose determines the poison." Anything can be harmful if you take too much of it. There have been several cases of people dying from drinking too much water. One of my patients developed mercury levels hundreds of times higher than normal from Indian ayurvedic medicines. Other people have developed vitamin D toxicity, requiring them to be hospitalized. The use of B vitamins has been associated with lung cancer, at least in men who smoke. One study estimated that the use of dietary supplements leads to 23,000 emergency department visits per year.

Another consequence of taking large quantities of these products is that they are often quite expensive. The vitamins and supplements industry is a big business. By some estimates, Americans spend $37 billion every year on supplements, a number that will grow larger in the next few years. Few of my patients have excess money to burn, and I suspect that their money could be put to better use. So, unless a specific deficiency is identified, I recommend that patients save their money.

56. What About Vitamin D?

One of the most intriguing aspects of MS is that it is much more common in areas that are far from the Equator. People who grow up near the Equator have a low risk of developing MS. The risk is determined by where a person spends the first 15 years of their life. Though this pattern has been known for many years, no one knows exactly why. One possible explanation has to deal with exposure to sunlight, which is necessary for the body to make vitamin D.

Vitamin D levels have been studied in patients with MS, and these patients have lower levels compared to healthy controls. One study found this to be the case during summer months specifically. This fluctuation in levels of vitamin D might be one reason why relapses have a seasonal variation, being more common in the spring and summer.

Despite this, it is too simplistic to say that low vitamin D levels cause MS. Rather, it is one of the many factors that interact to produce the disease in genetically vulnerable individuals.

The role for vitamin D supplementation once the diagnosis of MS has been made is controversial. Observational studies support the idea that MS patients with higher vitamin D levels have less disease activity. Other studies found that MS patients with higher vitamin D levels had a lower risk of new MRI lesions and lower disability. Higher vitamin D levels were associated with a lower relapse rate, but this was not statistically significant.

Another trial studied 49 patients and found that those who took high doses of vitamin D had their relapse rate cut by 41% compared with those who did not. Additionally, about double the percentage of patients receiving the high dose of vitamin D had no relapses at all compared with the control subjects. No safety concerns emerged.

Though these results are encouraging, the evidence that vitamin D supplementation fundamentally affects the course of MS is not that strong. One review paper examined five trials of vitamin D in MS. It found that "Of the five trials, four showed no effect of vitamin D on any outcome, and one showed a significant effect, namely upon reduction in the number of T1 enhancing lesions on brain magnetic resonance imaging." These results are not very impressive. Vitamin D supplementation was not entirely without side effects, and stomach upset was the most common symptom. In January 2018, the FDA rejected a company's claim that vitamin D could prevent MS. The FDA stated, "Based on the agency's review of the totality of publicly available scientific evidence, the FDA has concluded that there is no credible evidence of a relationship between intake of vitamin D and a reduced risk of MS."

Vitamin D obtained through supplements might function differently than vitamin D produced naturally via sunlight exposure. Indeed, one study found that in an animal model of MS, exposure to ultraviolet light, not vitamin D levels, impacted the disease. Perhaps getting direct sunlight exposure is more important than taking vitamin D supplements.

So, what is the upshot of these findings? Vitamin D supplements seem safe and they are inexpensive. However, the efficacy of vitamin D is only suggested at this time. Further research is needed to clarify the role of vitamin D in both preventing and treating MS.

57. What About Biotin?

Biotin, also called vitamin B7, has also been investigated as an MS treatment. In one study, 154 subjects with progressive MS received either high-dose biotin (also called MD1003) or a placebo for 1 year. Nearly 13% of those who received biotin showed improvement in disability while none on placebo did. A 36-month follow-up showed that biotin led to improved disability scores and walking ability. Another study investigated biotin in 93 patients with progressive visual worsening. It found that there was only slight improvement compared to placebo.

Unfortunately, at the end of 2017, the company developing high dose biotin for progressive MS abandoned attempts to get the medication approved in Europe. It was felt that the benefits were too small and its safety not clearly established. Still, some patients with progressive MS choose to get the medication from compounding pharmacies, hoping that it will slow down their disease progression. Importantly, biotin may interfere with several important lab tests, including the main test used to detect heart attacks

58.   *What About "Cure-Alls" in MS?*

Because MS is common, poorly understood, and incurable, every few years someone announces they have found a new "cure" for MS and patients are eager to believe it. Some of these "cures" are silly while others might be dangerous. When considering these quick fixes, I encourage all my patients to be cautious in seeking out unproven treatments, especially if they come with little scientific validation behind them. If a patient is thinking of trying out one of these marketed antidotes, they should talk to their neurologist first and be wary of companies selling products that might not live up to their expectations. Patients should be skeptical and be wary of supposed "miracle cures."

5 TREATING MS PART III: SYMPTOMS

59. What Are Symptomatic Treatments for MS?

Treating MS means not only trying to slow the disease itself, but also trying to alleviate its many symptoms. Importantly, many of the most distressing symptoms are "invisible." These include fatigue, pain, depression, cognitive dysfunction, sexual dysfunction, and urinary symptoms. Patients who appear to be well on the outside, might nonetheless be suffering from these symptoms. In one study, pain and depression caused the most distress to patients with MS.

Nearly all of the treatments to minimize these symptoms are not specific for MS, but they have been used for decades in MS patients. In contrast to the disease-modifying therapies, these symptomatic treatments work only if people *feel better*. As a result, their success is easier to judge. In addition to medications, nursing care, social work, occupational and physical therapy, and psychological counseling are all indispensable when treating patients with MS.

Finally, there is a tendency among patients and doctors alike to attribute every symptom an MS patient experiences to their MS. This is a mistake. Just because someone has MS does not relieve doctors of the responsibility of searching for other illnesses. When an MS patient complains of a symptom like fatigue, for example, it is still important to check for anemia and thyroid dysfunction. On several occasions, I have seen patients have other serious conditions in addition to their MS, such as blood clots in their extremities. Missing this diagnosis could lead to a fatal pulmonary embolus. Most of the time, when a patient has MS, their symptoms are caused by it. But patients and doctors alike need to be alert to the possibility that something else might be going on.

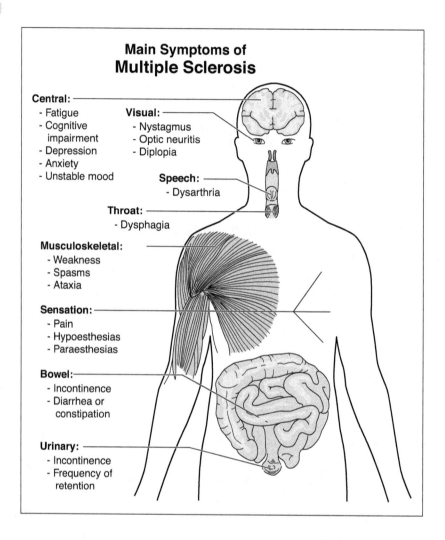

Main Symptoms of Multiple Sclerosis

Central:
- Fatigue
- Cognitive impairment
- Depression
- Anxiety
- Unstable mood

Visual:
- Nystagmus
- Optic neuritis
- Diplopia

Speech:
- Dysarthria

Throat:
- Dysphagia

Musculoskeletal:
- Weakness
- Spasms
- Ataxia

Sensation:
- Pain
- Hypoesthesias
- Paraesthesias

Bowel:
- Incontinence
- Diarrhea or constipation

Urinary:
- Incontinence
- Frequency of retention

FATIGUE: Fatigue is both one of the most common and most disabling symptoms in MS. It is also one of the major factors limiting employment. We all lead busy lives, but the fatigue in MS is often more disabling than the normal fatigue of everyday life.

The best intervention to fight fatigue is to get enough rest, and the best way to get enough rest is to practice good sleep hygiene. Sleep hygiene describes habits and behaviors that promote proper sleep, using free, risk-free behavioral interventions. While many of these interventions are "common sense," surprisingly few people practice good sleep hygiene. For some people, learning how to sleep properly is a skill that take time and practice to master, but the rewards can be worth the effort. There is also nothing magical about 8 hours of sleep. Some people need more, and some people need less. Here are some key techniques of sleep hygiene.

Maintain a Regular Sleep Routine
- As much as possible, people try to fall asleep and wake up at the same time every night, even on the weekends.
- Have a bedtime routine of a warm bath or quiet reading.

Make Your Bedroom Comfortable and Quiet
- As much as possible, make your room dark, quiet, and cool. Even a charging phone can emit enough light to disrupt some people's sleep.
- If you live in a noisy city, a white noise machine can be used to block out the honking and sirens.

Use the Bed for Sleep and Sex
- Your bed should be associated only with sleep and sex. Don't watch TV, goof off on the Internet, or play video games in bed. These behaviors will make you associate your bed with wakefulness.

Avoid Naps if Possible
- Some patients find that naps are a necessary part of their day. If this is the case, then all attempts should be made to avoid napping late in the afternoon, which will make it difficult to fall asleep at night. Just like going to sleep at night, naps should be taken at the same time daily. Also, naps should not be longer than 45 minutes.

Don't Remain in Bed if You Have Trouble Sleeping
- If you have trouble sleeping, don't toss and turn in bed. You cannot "force" yourself to sleep. If you are still not asleep after 20 minutes, sit quietly in a dark room until you are ready to fall asleep.
- If you find yourself staring at the clock while in bed, hide the clock.

Go to the Bathroom Before Bed
- Even if you don't have to, force yourself to go to the bathroom before bed. This will minimize the chances that you have to get up and go in the middle of the night.

Don't Drink Caffeine or Take Stimulant Medications in the Afternoon and Evening
- If you drink caffeine or take a stimulant medication, the effects can last for many hours, even if you are not consciously aware of them. For this reason, these substances should only be used in the morning.

Don't Rely on Sleep Medications

▓ Some people reach a point where they cannot sleep without medications. The best way to avoid this is not to start them in the first place or to use them as infrequently as possible.

Exercise 3-6 Hours Before Bedtime

▓ Exercise is important, but don't do it right before you try to fall asleep.

A referral to a sleep center may be indicated for some patients. For many patients, fatigue remains a significant problem even after a full night's sleep. For such individuals, medications to promote alertness may be required. Several options exist, including Amantadine, Provigil, and Nuvigil, as well as stimulants such as Adderall and Ritalin. Some patients choose to take these medications only on busy days, avoiding them on the weekends. Unfortunately, formal evidence that these treatments help in MS is lacking and one study of Provigil found it did not relieve fatigue more than placebo.

PAIN: Unfortunately, pain is common in MS. Pain directly due to MS is usually described as a burning, electrical sensation in the hands and feet or a "hugging," band-like" sensation around the torso. These symptoms of "nerve pain" are most commonly due to lesions in the spinal cord and is most commonly treated with antiepileptic medications such as gabapentin and Lyrica, or antidepressant medications such as Cymbalta and Elavil. In severe cases, opioids are considered to make patients more comfortable, but due to their serious side effects, they are only used when absolutely necessary. Medical marijuana is also an option.

Some patients may develop a severe, electrical pain to one side of their face, called trigeminal neuralgia. This can usually be controlled with an antiepileptic medication called Tegretol, which is the medication of choice for this diagnosis. However, in some cases neurosurgical procedures may be required to treat the pain.

Patients with difficult to treat pain may benefit from a referral to a pain management specialist. Not surprisingly, there is a strong relationship between pain and depression in MS, and it is important to try to treat both of these.

Other aspects of MS, such as reduced mobility, may indirectly lead to pain. This is best treated with physical and occupational therapy. Of course, pain is common in many people without MS, and doctors should be careful not to prematurely ascribe someone's pain to their MS without investigating other potential causes. In addition to medications, targeted injection therapy can be used for certain types of non-MS related pain. Conditions that may respond to this treatment include nerve root impingement in the neck or lower back, chronic migraine, and arthritis in joints such as the knee and hip.

NYSTAGMUS: Nystagmus refers to rapid, repetitive, uncontrolled eye movements. Such movements are common in MS and can cause visual disturbances, vertigo, and trouble reading. Though it can be difficult to treat, there is some evidence that gabapentin and memantine (a medication used in Alzheimer's disease) can be helpful in treating this symptom. Other medications, such as Baclofen (lioresal) and Ampyra (4-aminopyridine) may be helpful as well, depending on the type of nystagmus.

SPASTICITY: Spasticity is a condition in which certain muscles are continuously contracted, resulting in stiffness and tightness. It is caused by damage to the part of the brain or spinal cord that controls voluntary movement. *Spasticity* can make walking difficult, cause fatigue and pain, and interrupt sleep. The treatment of spasticity is multifactorial.

- If smaller muscles such as those of the hand are stiff, patients may get relief from periodic injections of Botox (botulinum toxin).

- For larger muscles, stretching exercises may help to temporarily alleviate mild spasticity.

- When stretching is not effective, neurologists may recommend a pill such as Baclofen. Baclofen may be started at a low dose and slowly increased until maximum benefit is achieved. If the dose is too high it may cause the muscles to relax too much, making it difficult to stand and walk. Side effects include excessive weakness, sedation, dizziness, and confusion. Zanaflex (tizanidine) is another pill that can be used alone or in addition to Baclofen when Baclofen on its own is not enough to control spasticity. Side effects of Zanaflex include sleepiness, dry mouth, weakness, liver toxicity, and orthostatic hypotension (dizziness when standing from a seated and lying position).

- If patients require still more medication, an intrathecal Baclofen pump is an option. The pump delivers a highly concentrated liquid Baclofen directly to the spinal canal where it reduces spasticity. It looks similar to a hockey puck and is computerized. It is placed under the skin in the abdominal area in a simple surgical procedure. While it can be felt, it is not visible.

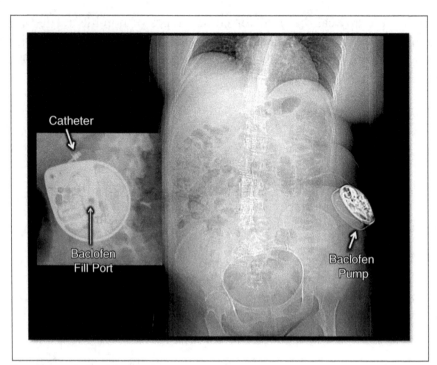

Two views of a Baclofen pump.

In the image, you can see the Baclofen fill port. A clinician can easily access this port to refill the pump with Baclofen when needed, which is usually every couple of months. The catheter itself looks like string. It is attached to the pump and threaded to the spinal canal where it will slowly dispense Baclofen via the catheter. The amount of Baclofen dispensed can be changed by placing a magnet over the pump and changing the computer settings.

In order to determine if a person is a good candidate for a Baclofen pump, an appointment is scheduled for a trial injection. On this day, the patient does not take any anti-spasticity medications. A physical therapist then assesses the amount of spasticity the patient has. A physician then numbs an area of the spine and a small amount of Baclofen is injected into the spinal canal. The physical therapist then measures the individual's spasticity again and asks the patient whether they notice a benefit. If everyone agrees that it was beneficial, a date for surgery is made to implant the pump. Of course, if there is a problem, the pump can be removed at any time.

MENTAL HEALTH: The most common mental health issues in MS are depression and anxiety. Of course other psychiatric conditions, such as bipolar disorder, schizophrenia, substance abuse, obsessive-compulsive disorder, and eating disorders occur in MS patients but are less often the focus of treatment. About 50% of MS patients develop major depression over the course of their lives, a rate two to five times higher than in the general population. At any moment one third of MS patients may suffer from depression.

In one study, two questions were enough to diagnose depression in nearly all MS patients with this disorder.

- During the past month, have you often been bothered by feeling down, depressed, or hopeless?
- During the past month, have you often been bothered by little interest or pleasure in doing things?

Up to 25% of MS patients may contemplate suicide. Risk factors for suicide are the presence of severe depression, social isolation, and substance abuse. While only a minority of suicidal patients will act on these thoughts, completed suicide is more common in individuals with MS. Young men within the first 5 years of diagnosis have the highest risk.

Anxiety is common in MS as well. The unpredictable course of MS makes it a "perfect" disease to cause anxiety. One of my patients was stabbed in the back and will never walk again. But because there is no uncertainty about his condition, he is psychiatrically very healthy. In contrast, many MS patients live in a constant state of anxiety as they ponder what their future holds. The causes of depression in MS are multifactorial. A number of factors have been linked to depression in MS: uncertainty, feelings of helplessness, reduced enjoyment of recreational activities, poor quality of social relationships, high levels of stress, and the adoption of particular maladaptive coping strategies. Importantly, there is no evidence that depression precedes MS, nor is there evidence that a single lesion causes depression.

Of course, depression is common in the general population and many patients have extraordinarily stressful lives independent of their MS. Some patients were depressed before they were diagnosed with MS and would remain so if the cure for MS was found tomorrow. There is little evidence to support the dogma that medications used to treat MS, specifically the interferons, cause depression. However, the interferons should be used in caution in patients with a history of severe depression.

The treatment of depression in MS is similar to the treatment of depression in general. Studies of antidepressants in MS have been small, short in duration, and uncontrolled. Many of the medications used to treat depression also help with anxiety.

Unfortunately, few depressed patients respond to medication alone. As such, psychotherapy and psychosocial interventions are usually the most important components of treating depression. There is good evidence that such interventions effectively treat a wide range of psychiatric symptoms in MS. There are several online resources to help patients find a therapist.

Social isolation, though hard to quantify, is the biggest enemy of many MS patients. Support groups may be very valuable for those that feel they are becoming isolated. Support groups offer patients an opportunity to talk to other people who can understand their symptoms in a way someone without MS cannot. The Multiple Sclerosis Society can help connect patients to support groups near where they live.

When all else fails, electroconvulsive therapy (ECT) can be used in severely depressed, suicidal patients. The available data suggest that ECT is safe and effective in MS.

PSEUDOBULBAR PALSY: Some patients, usually those with longstanding MS and cognitive impairment, develop a symptom called pseudobulbar palsy, which is characterized by uncontrolled episodes of crying or laughing. It can be treated with Neudexta, a combination of dextromethorphan and quinidine.

HEAT INTOLERANCE: The tendency of MS symptoms to worsen when body temperature increases has been noted for over 100 years. This is known as Uthoff's phenomenon, after an ophthalmologist who noticed that the symptoms in patients with optic neuritis tended to become worse as their body temperature rose. Elevated body temperatures slow down conduction in the nerves, explaining why old MS symptoms worsen with heat. In fact, prior to MRIs, patients suspected of having MS were sometimes placed in warm baths to bring out their symptoms as a part of the diagnosis.

It is very common for patients to experience the transient return of prior neurological symptoms when they are in a hot shower or outside on a hot day. Often MS patients don't experience the recurrence of specific neurological symptoms such as numbness or visual loss, but rather an overwhelming sense of fatigue and malaise. Of course, no one wants to do anything other than sit in front of a powerful air conditioner when it is 100 degrees outside, but for many MS patients this desire to escape the heat is magnified.

Heat is not dangerous for MS and does not cause new symptoms or relapses. Rather, it may cause old, partially healed symptoms of MS to return. So, MS patients should not be afraid of the sun or a hot shower, but they should know that they might be sensitive to the heat and should not over-exert themselves in the summer sun.

Heat intolerance is best treated with common-sense measures, such as staying in the shade and carrying cool water on hot days. Cooling vests that hold small ice packets are also available. These are generously given for free by the Multiple Sclerosis Association of America. The National Multiple Sclerosis Society also offers vouchers to help patients buy air conditioners.

TROUBLE WALKING: Walking difficulties are some of the most common and disabling symptoms of MS. Ampyra (dalfampridine) is used to improve walking speed in patients with MS. It is a pill that is taken twice a day and is the only symptomatic treatment that is specific to MS. It works by blocking potassium channels in axons, thereby improving nerve conduction in injured areas of the brain and spinal cord. Prior to its approval by the FDA in 2010, dalfampridine was available through compounding pharmacies. Previously, it was called fampridine or 4-aminopyridine (4AP).

So, what does Ampyra really do? In clinical studies, patients who took it had improvement in their walking speed (as measured on a 25-foot walk) four times as often as those who took placebo. Responders to Ampyra were defined as patients whose walking speed was faster on at least three of four on-treatment visits than their fastest speed at any of five off-treatment visits. Ampyra resulted in an approximately 25% increase in walking speed in about 40% of patients, as well as improved leg strength. The benefits of Ampyra seem to be maintained over several years. Ampyra may also be helpful in other domains as well, such as vision, cognition, and arm strength, but this has not been formally proven. Unfortunately, Ampyra does not work for everybody. In the clinical trials, 60% of patients did not respond to the medicine.

Ampyra is generally very safe. In clinical trials, no serious adverse effects were noted in the patients who took Ampyra when compared to those who took placebo. At higher doses than 10 mg twice daily (studied in other trials), Ampyra was associated with seizures. The medication should, therefore, not be used in patients with a history of seizures or in anyone with kidney disease, as the medicine might build up to toxic levels. In the clinical trials, subjects who took the medicine reported more symptoms consistent with a urinary tract infection compared to those who received placebo.

Certainly, it is wonderful to have a generally safe pill that can help with a potentially disabling symptom of MS. I tell patients starting Ampyra that it is unlikely to be a miracle, but it certainly may help them. While some patients say it has made a huge impact in their lives, my experience is similar to that of the trials---many patients do not feel significantly different on the medication. High doses of amantadine, an older antiviral medication that is also used in Parkinson's disease, has also shown promise to improve walking speed in small trials. Further studies are ongoing.

Another way to improve walking is a device that gives an electrical signal to the nerve that lifts up the foot or knee. This device is worn on the leg and is useful in patients who have a foot drop or have trouble straightening their knee. Several companies make the device, including WalkAide and Bioness. While the device is safe and can be very helpful, its main drawback is its price.

LET'S TALK ABOUT SEX, BABY: Sexual arousal is a combination of our emotions, energy level, and all of our senses. Unfortunately, MS can affect nearly all aspects of sexuality, and sexual dysfunction is common in MS. In one survey, 63% of people with MS reported decreased sexual activity. Another survey found that sexual dysfunction affects 91% of men and 72% of women with MS. Sexual dysfunction is a combination of both physical and emotional factors. The physical factors can be directly due to injury to the central nervous system or due to secondary symptoms such as stiffness and loss of mobility.

Physical Factors
- Decreased libido
- Genital numbness, pain, increased sensitivity
- Difficulty or inability to maintain erection
- Decreased vaginal lubrication
- Decreased vaginal muscle tone
- Ejaculation difficulty
- Problems having an orgasm
- Difficulty moving

Emotional Factors
- Depression, anxiety, and anger
- Stress of living with MS (and life in general)
- Anger

▦ Low self-esteem

▦ Feeling undesirable

▦ Loss of spontaneity

Erectile dysfunction is by far the most common problem for men. Other problems include reduced sensation and difficulty achieving ejaculation. Treatment options include medications for erectile dysfunction such as Viagra, Levitra, and Cialis. Other treatment options include injectable medications that increase blood flow in the penis, inserting a small suppository into the penis to enhance blood flow, penile implants, or the use of vacuum devices and penile pumps to help achieve an erection. Obviously, these must be done under the care of a qualified urologist. Penile injections need to be properly taught and supervised to avoid long-lasting erections (called priapism) that can damage the penis tissue.

Women may experience reduced vaginal sensation, vaginal dryness, or painfully heightened sensation. Vaginal dryness can be relieved by using liquid or jellied, water-soluble personal lubricants. It is a common mistake to use too little of these products. Women may also benefit from Eros Therapy, which is a hand-held device used to improve blood flow to the clitoris and genitalia, increasing orgasms and vaginal lubrication. Wrapping a bag of frozen peas in a cloth and holding this around the painful area can help with vaginal pain. Certain products, such as Vagi-Kool, can also be used for this purpose.

All patients with sexual dysfunction should periodically review their medications with their neurologist. Some medications, especially antidepressants, can cause loss of libido. Others can cause fatigue, making sexual arousal difficult.

Counseling with a sexual therapist can also be helpful in addressing other issues that may interfere with sex. Remember, an MS diagnosis does not mean that your sexual life is terminated as several treatments are available to help with this important matter.

BLADDER DYSFUNCTION: Over 75% of MS patients will experience some bladder dysfunction. The symptoms appear on average 6 to 8 years after diagnosis. The types and severity of these problems depend upon the location of injury to the central nervous system, the duration of the MS, and the overall degree of neurological disability. Not surprisingly, more severe urinary problems are seen in wheelchair-bound patients.

Bladder dysfunction is of concern for two reasons. Firstly, it might significantly impair quality of life, especially when urinary incontinence is present. Secondly, it may cause urinary tract infections, urinary stones, or kidney failure. In severe situations, these might be life-threatening. For these reasons, your doctors should ask about urinary symptoms and you should not hesitate to mention them yourself. They may order some basic blood tests to evaluate your kidney function and a urinary tract ultrasound looking for kidney abnormalities and incomplete bladder emptying.

Several different urinary symptoms might occur with MS, but the most common are those called overactive bladder symptoms. These symptoms are due to bladder spasms that make it difficult for the bladder to hold urine. Specific symptoms include:

- *Urgency:* An urgent desire to void that cannot be delayed and can cause urine leakage.

- *Frequency:* Having to urinate multiple times during the day.

- *Nocturia:* Waking at night to urinate.

Another common issue in MS is difficult voiding, meaning patients are unable to completely empty their bladders. As the bladder and bowel share nerves, constipation or fecal incontinence may accompany bladder dysfunction.

If the urinary symptoms are not severe and there are no urological complications, a neurologist or primary care physician can manage them using the first-line conservative measures. When symptoms are not relieved by these treatments or there are urinary complications, a referral to a neuro-urologist is appropriate. A neuro-urologist specializes in managing urinary dysfunction due to neurological diseases, and will likely require additional testing. The most common test is called urodynamic testing. During this test, small catheters are inserted into the bladder and rectum to record the bladder and abdominal pressure. This helps to precisely understand the mechanism of bladder dysfunction and to check that the bladder pressure is not too high, which is a risky urinary situation. Ultimately this test will help to select the most appropriate treatment option.

Several options are now available to treat MS-related urinary problems. The first option is behavioral therapy. For bladder-holding issues, this encompasses:

- *Pelvic floor muscle training/Kegel exercise:* These exercises involve contractions of pelvic floor muscles to calm down bladder spasms.

- *Bladder training:* Voluntarily holding on to urine for increasingly longer periods.

■   *Fluid intake management:* Diminishing fluid intake after 6 P.M can reduce nocturia, as can cutting down on fluids that might irritate the bladder such as alcohol, coffee, and tea.

Those general measures always help at least partly but are insufficient in most MS patients. Medications are usually the second-line treatment for bladder-holding issues. The most commonly prescribed medications are a class of medications called anticholinergics. Examples include Detrol (tolterodine), Ditropan (oxybutynin), Sanctura (trospium), Enablex (darifenacin), Toviaz (fesoterodine), and Vesicare (solifenacin). Ditropan is also available as a transdermal patch. The main side effects of these medications are mostly dry mouth and constipation. A newer medication called Myrbetriq (mirabegron) is increasingly prescribed in MS as it largely avoids these side effects. A hormone called desmopressin or antidiuretic hormone can be taken at bedtime for patients who awaken during the night to urinate. If medications fail to treat urgent desires to void, the next step is usually Botox injections into the bladder. This is done in the office under local anesthesia once or twice a year to relax the muscles of the bladder.

Neuromodulation is another option in selected patients. This uses electrical stimulation emanating from a small needle inserted at the ankle or a pacemaker inserted directly to the bladder nerves at the lower back. This helps modulate communication between the central nervous system and the bladder.

For bladder emptying issues, behavioral therapy involves voiding at regularly scheduled times and double-voiding, which lessens the amount of urine left into the bladder. In most cases of voiding problems, medications called alpha-blockers are used to relax the urinary sphincter and facilitate bladder emptying.

If bladder emptying problems are more severe, there may be a high volume of urine left in the bladder after urination. In this situation intermittent self-catheterization might be indicated. This involves inserting a small catheter into the urethra to completely drain the bladder. This will not only relieve urinary symptoms and keep people dry, it will also protect their kidneys from potentially severe complications. Most patients are naturally intimidated by this option, but after learning more about it, most patients feel it will make their lives easier and better. A clear distinction has to be made between this self-catheterization and the permanent, indwelling urethral catheters that were used with MS patients in the past. Those indwelling catheters should not be used anymore as they carry very high risks of urinary tract infections, urethral injuries, and, in the long-run, even bladder cancer.

In patients with advanced neurological impairment, a suprapubic tube can be used to permanently drain the bladder. This tube is placed at the lower part of the abdomen, and it collects urine in a small bag that is hidden under clothing. When these options fail, a surgical procedure called urinary diversion or ileal conduit may be offered. This involves creating a hole to directly collect the urine in a pouch at the abdominal wall level. The bag containing the urine is changed every 3 to 7 days. Although it is a last resort, several studies have shown that this improves the quality of life and helps protect the kidneys in patients with advanced MS and severe bladder dysfunction.

Urinary tract infections are also a common problem in MS patients. These fall into two categories: (a) bladder infections with urinary symptoms such as burning and bladder pain, and (b) kidney or prostate infections with more serious symptoms such as fever, fatigue, and chills. Both of these are treated with antibiotics after a urine sample is collected. The treatment for bladder infections is shorter and done outside the hospital, while kidney or prostate infections are more serious and often require hospitalization with IV antibiotics. A positive urine culture does not mean that someone has a urinary tract infection, however. Most people, especially those with MS, have bacteria in their bladder permanently that does not cause symptoms. This is called asymptomatic colonization. In this situation no antibiotics are required. Treatment is only required for a positive urine culture if there are symptoms.

In summary, urinary problems are common in MS and can cause serious dysfunction. However, multiple options are available to manage them and to minimize their impact on your health and life.

COGNITION: Cognitive dysfunction refers to any decline in thinking ability. This includes difficulty with concentration, learning or remembering information, finding the right words when speaking, and making proper decisions. Cognitive dysfunction is very common in MS, affecting more than 70% of all patients. Slowed information processing is usually the first type of cognitive dysfunction to be experienced in patients with MS.

While cognitive dysfunction is easy to detect in some patients, it may go unnoticed in patients with a high overall level of functioning. To establish a baseline and monitor for progression, a neuropsychological evaluation may be beneficial. While often troublesome, cognitive dysfunction in MS is usually milder than in other brain diseases and typically does not lead to a rapid decline. At times, however, it can be disabling enough to lead to unemployment and dependence on caregivers. Rarely, it can be the main symptom of MS.

The first step in dealing with cognitive dysfunction is to address any treatable factors other than MS itself. These include psychiatric disorders, medication side effects, and fatigue. Although the disease-modifying medications used in MS may slow the progression of cognitive decline, at present there are no drugs that directly improve cognition. Therefore, the most important way to preserve cognition is to maintain overall physical health. A healthy diet and regular exercise can help both the body and mind function at their best. There is some evidence that aerobic exercise is helpful specifically for cognitive dysfunction in MS.

There is also truth to the saying "Use or it or lose it." Engaging in cognitively challenging activities on a daily basis can be helpful. Studies have shown that cognitive rehabilitation or remediation can have a modest benefit in MS. This includes both individual training programs as well as online "brain training" programs. These can improve processing speed, and a beneficial effect has been documented specifically in MS. Research has also suggested that a meditation program called mindfulness may lead to cognitive benefit. As with the brain training programs, more is better, with the suggestion of daily practice for up to an hour each day leading to the best results.

Cognitive remediation may assist in providing compensatory strategies to help improve daily functioning. Specific examples include:

- Put all of your important belongings, such as your money, phone, and keys in one location in your house.

- Use your phone as a second brain. Most people have smart phones that can remind them of appointments and when to take medications. It can also store to-do lists and other important information.

- Use memory techniques. People are more likely to remember things if they see them, hear them, write them, and read them. Personally, I manage to remember my keys, wallet, and phone most days because I sing a little jingle before I leave the house.

- Do one activity at a time. Listening to the radio or music when trying to make plans can be distracting. If you are trying to remember something important, try to make that the focus of your attention.

- Take it easy on yourself. Everyone forgets things now and then. People with MS often fear that normal forgetfulness is a sign of declining cognitive skills.

TREMOR: A tremor is a rhythmic back-and-forth oscillation of muscles. In MS, tremors are most often due to pathology of the cerebellum. The tremor is usually an action tremor, meaning that it is worse when patients move their arms to reach for an object. Unfortunately, it is one of the most disabling symptoms for some patients and the most difficult to treat. Medications that are used to try to reduce tremors include antiepileptic medications, Propranolol®, and Klonopin. A small study found that Botox was effective as well. In severe situations, some patients may benefit from a neurosurgical procedure called deep brain stimulation, which is mostly used in Parkinson's disease. Occupational therapy can be invaluable in helping patients maximize their function despite a tremor.

60. What About Marijuana?

The use of marijuana is common in MS, with estimates of use ranging from 20% to 60%. Tetrahydrocannabinol (THC) and cannabidiol (CBD) are the main active ingredients. THC is what gets people "high," while CBD is non-intoxicating. Although some people proclaim that marijuana is a miracle cure-all, this is not the case. There is no evidence that it impacts the course of MS. One study of 498 subjects found that oral dronabinol (a form of THC) had no impact in patients with progressive MS. Cannabinoids do have a role as symptomatic therapy. They have been shown to be useful to treat pain and stiffness in MS. Research shows that there is a "modest" effect on these parameters.

Of course, access to legal cannabinoids varies widely from state to state and the cost can be prohibitive for some patients. As such, many people choose to buy non-prescription marijuana. However, the price to be paid, and this is no surprise, is that marijuana can impact cognition in patients with MS. Heavy users of marijuana perform worse on cognitive tests compared to non-users. Like any medication, the risks and benefits of marijuana need to be weighed against each other.

MS Symptoms and Possible Treatments

Symptom	Treatments
Fatigue	Provigil, Nuvigil, Amantadine, Stimulants, Improved Sleep Hygiene
Pain	NSAIDs, Antiepileptics, Antidepressants, Medical Marijuana, Surgery For Trigeminal Neuralgia, Opioids
Nystagmus	Baclofen, Klonopin, Gabapentin, Memantine

(continued)

Symptom	Treatments
Spasticity	Baclofen (orally or via intrathecal pump), Zanaflex, Benzodiazepines, Botox
Mental Health	SSRIs, SNRIs, Wellbutrin, Psychotherapy, Group Therapy
Pseudobulbar Palsy	Nuedexta
Heat Intolerance	Cooling Vests
Trouble Walking	Ampyra, Physical Therapy, WalkAide/Bioness Devices
Sexual dysfunction for women	Vagi-Kool, Eros Therapy, lubricants
Sexual dysfunction for men	Viagra, Levitra, and Cialis, Injectable Medications Penile Implants, Inflatable Devices
Bladder dysfunction	Anticholinergic Medications, Desmopressin, Botox, Self-Catheterization, Suprapubic Tube
Cognition	Cognitive Rehabilitation, BrainHQ
Tremor	Antiepileptics, Propranolol, Klonopin, Botox, Deep Brain Stimulation

61. What Is Polypharmacy?

It is clear there are many medications to minimize the symptoms of MS. All of them come with possible side effects, and patients need to be careful of something called polypharmacy. This is a fancy way of saying "too many medications." Some patients are on a large number of medications, and it is difficult to tell if they are helping them more than they are hurting them. Sometimes patients are on medications to counteract the side effects of other medications! For example, some patients are on medications that make them tired, so they need something to wake them up. Polypharmacy is not just a waste of money; it increases the risk of dangerous drug interactions or side effects. Taking too many medications can be dangerous, especially in older or vulnerable patients.

Because polypharamcy can increase risk, it is important that MS patients always bring a list of their medications to their visit with their neurologist. Though computer systems should have this list, they do not always accurately reflect what patients actually take. At least once per year, patients should review all of their medications with their neurologist to determine which ones may be unnecessary. Also, whenever possible, neurologists should try to "kill two birds with one stone" and use one medication for two or more symptoms. Often, a medication can be used for more than one purpose. For example, if a patient suffers from depression and pain, Cymbalta can help with both of these symptoms.

62. What Is the Role of Physical Therapy in MS?

Physical therapists are licensed health care professionals who help patients improve or restore their mobility with the ultimate goal of improving or restoring their quality of life. More than 91% of all persons with MS report difficulty with body movements and walking. Physical therapists examine, evaluate, and treat patients whose conditions limit their ability to move and function. They are crucial members of the health care team, addressing the rehabilitation needs of patients with MS, working with them to maintain, restore, or improve their functional abilities.

During an initial physical therapy visit, patients will undergo a thorough examination. The examination will start with an interview, during which the physical therapist will get to know the patient better and ensure that their concerns are addressed. The physical therapist will ask about the patient's health, the specific reasons they are seeking services, and their goals for physical therapy. The physical therapist will also ask about the patient's home, work, health habits, activity level, as well as leisure and recreational activities. The goal is to make sure the whole person is considered and not just someone's medical condition. Following the interview, the physical therapist will perform tests to measure strength, flexibility, balance, endurance, and coordination. The physical therapist will also observe movements, such as walking, how the patient gets in and out of a chair, how they go up and down stairs, and any other activities that are meaningful to the patient.

Once the physical therapist has identified areas of strength and weakness, the physical therapist will develop an individualized plan of care, which will include specific interventions. The main goal of treatment is to improve or maintain someone's ability to perform their daily tasks and activities. An important aspect of any physical therapy intervention will be education. More specifically, the physical therapist teaches patients special exercises to do at home. Patients might also learn new techniques to perform activities. These techniques might help minimize fatigue, falls, or injuries, and optimize independence. The physical therapist will also evaluate the need for special equipment, such as canes or walkers, which can enable people to move safely.

The physical therapist will monitor a patient's progress and work with them to plan for their discharge from physical therapy. They will also give patients specific instructions on what to do after discharge. Like most things in life, patients will get out of therapy as much as they put in. Sufficient effort as agreed upon between patients and their physical therapist is necessary to maximize the benefits from each session. The main goal is to assist people in resuming their roles at home, at work, and in their community.

63. What Is the Role of Occupational Therapy in MS?

The purpose of occupational therapy is to improve an individual's independence and safety in their daily activities. This includes everything from taking a shower to feeding oneself, to meal preparation and performing work-related tasks. This improvement can be achieved through a hybrid of both restorative and compensatory approaches. For example, if a patient is experiencing issues buttoning a shirt, an occupational therapist would evaluate and work with them to improve their active range of motion, fine motor coordination, and sensory deficits. An occupational therapist may also educate the patient on adaptive equipment, body mechanics principles, and energy conservation strategies to improve their functionality.

One of the primary goals of occupational therapy is to ensure safety for patients when getting in and out of their home. Occupational therapists may spend treatment sessions addressing safety awareness as well as educating patients on fall prevention, energy conservation, and problem-solving techniques to employ during self-care and household tasks. Interventions may include addressing tasks such as grocery shopping, laundry, or utilizing public transportation. An occupational therapist may recommend and train an individual in use of durable medical equipment (such as grab bars and shower chairs) and recommend home modifications to prevent falls and to improve safety and independence during self-care tasks. At times, an occupational therapist may visit a patient's house to make sure proper equipment is installed and fall risks are minimized.

If a patient is having difficulty with medication adherence, an occupational therapist would further assess and treat any relevant cognitive, physical, visual, or behavioral deficits. In addition to trying to restore function, an occupational therapist might work with the patient to help develop compensatory tools to deal with medication. This may include physically modifying a medication bottle and/or the environment, prescribing a medication tracking application, or a specific pillbox.

If a patient with MS experiences changes in communication abilities and/or active movement in their upper or lower body, they may benefit from being seen by an occupational therapist who can prescribe and train them in the use of assistive technologies. These include adaptive keyboards, software, and/or modifications to improve ease when using a computer, TV remote, phone, or lights.

If a patient is experiencing MS-related symptoms or having increasing difficulty with any of their daily activities or roles, it is best to discuss these issues with their neurologist about whether or not they could benefit from an occupational therapy referral. By addressing each issue from multiple angles, a patient may demonstrate progress toward each functional goal.

64. What Mobility Assistive Devices Are Available?

Weakness, poor balance, fatigue, and pain are common symptoms in MS. All of these can affect a patient's ability to walk, limiting their independence. A mobility evaluation is essential for patients who are a fall risk or have difficulty participating in outside activities. This specialty evaluation is conducted by an occupational or physical therapist. It helps determine if a mobility device can reduce a patient's fall risk and increase their independence. There are several types of mobility assistive devices commonly used by patients with MS:

ORTHOTICS: Orthotics and braces anchor and align the knees and ankles to minimize walking difficulties. An example includes an ankle-foot orthosis, which helps to control the position and motion of the ankle to compensate for weakness.

CANES/CRUTCHES: There is a wide variety of canes, many of which can adjust in height or fold to fit in a purse or bag. Some have a base that can stand on its own, allowing patients to let the cane go without it falling over. Some crutches anchor onto the elbow, while others fit under the shoulder.

WALKERS: Walkers provide a wide base of support, providing extra stability. Rollators are a type of walker with wheels, hand breaks, and a seat. Many have a basket that allows patients to transport their belongings.

MANUAL WHEELCHAIR: Patients move manual wheelchairs with their arms and feet. They can also be pushed by caregivers. Some fold easily into the trunk of a vehicle. Others do not fold, and these have better rolling performance. Wheelchair weight varies from standard-weight to light-weight. A variety of seat cushions and back supports are available to account for different postures and to maximize patient comfort. Manual wheelchairs need to be properly sized by an expert. If they are too wide or if the wheels are too far part, it can be difficult for patients to propel themselves, causing shoulder pain and fatigue.

POWER WHEELCHAIR: Power wheelchairs are technologically sophisticated chairs that can offer certain patients greater independence and freedom than manual wheelchairs. They have a motor and a drive control, which is usually a hand-operated joystick. They can be adapted so patients can use switches or alternate controls. Patients who do not have use of their hands can steer the chair with their head or even their breath. There are different types of frames depending on the location of the drive wheels.

Patients can also elevate the seat to help transfer on and off the chair and reach for objects overhead. The leg rest can elevate to minimize leg pain and swelling. Different types of seating functions are available that allow patients to shift their weight and move their bodies to maximize comfort and mobility.

Power wheelchairs require a ramp to enter spaces with barriers, such as stairs. Patients need houses with wide doorways and corridors to use the wheelchair at home. Their motors and batteries also need to be charged.

SCOOTERS: Scooters are controlled by moving a tiller that is similar to a bicycle. Patients must have some mobility, as they have to be able to step-up onto a platform to sit. Because they are difficult to maneuver and to operate indoors and in tight spaces, they are most useful for outdoor and long-distance mobility. Some scooters can be taken apart to fit in a vehicle.

Payment for wheelchairs and scooters varies based on whether patients have a commercial insurance, Medicare, or Medicaid. Getting insurance approval often takes many months. Patients should be proactive and begin the process of getting insurance approval as soon they decide to get a mobility device. The National Multiple Sclerosis Society has funds available to help patients purchase and repair mobility devices, as well as to modify their homes to make them wheelchair-accessible.

6 LIFESTYLE AND MS

65. What Lifestyle Changes Should I Make?

It is natural for patients with MS to do everything they can to improve their health. Patients often ask what they can do to improve the course of their disease. Other than taking medications and certain lifestyle adjustments that will be discussed, there is not much to be done. This may seem disempowering, but I hope this is not the case. It is my firm belief that most patients should lead the life they were living before they had the disease. So, if they enjoyed staying out late, eating a nice meal, having a few beers, and drinking coffee in the morning, I don't want MS to change that. Patients with MS should not feel that they are delicate glass flowers that will shatter if they do something "wrong." This attitude is profoundly disempowering to patients, causing them to blame themselves for their disease and live in fear of pleasurable activities.

66. What Is the Best Thing I Can Do for My Health?

People with MS are not a different species. Most will live a normal lifespan and most will die of the same things that kill everyone else: heart disease, cancer, and stroke. To a large degree, these killers can be modified through a healthy lifestyle. So, *just like everyone else*, here are the most important things for people with MS to do:

- **Exercise:** Any movement is beneficial. While vigorous exercise might not be possible for all MS patients, almost everyone can do some exercise. If MS is destined to take away 10% of someone's strength, they will be better off if they start out from a strong baseline. Physical and occupational therapy can be very helpful in this regard.

- **Eat fresh fruits and vegetables while minimizing junk food:** Everyone knows that healthy eating is a key to a healthy life. While I am not convinced that a healthy diet can fundamentally alter the course of

MS (I discuss this in the next section), a healthy diet can lower the risk of cardiovascular disease, which is the top killer of Americans. There is no reason to be afraid of pizza and ice cream now and then, just don't make them a daily part of your life.

- **Get enough sleep:** Due to pain, stiffness, and bladder-control issues, patients with MS may have more trouble sleeping. Also, some of the medications used to treat fatigue in MS can interfere with sleep if they are taken late in the day. However, the biggest problem with sleep is that most people just don't get enough of it. We are all up too late at night, watching TV or playing on our phones. However, sleep deprivation can lead to fatigue, irritability, and a large number of other health problems. Getting enough sleep is one of the keys to good health.

- **Don't isolate yourself:** For many of my patients, social isolation is their single biggest obstacle to enjoying life. Whether you have MS or not, it's important to enjoy life, and surround yourself with family and friends. Of course, not everyone has a large, supportive family or a large group of friends to help them. Support groups can be very valuable for people without this traditional base of support.

- **Stop smoking and drink in moderation:** I know it's easier said than done, but there is no question that quitting is the best thing smokers can do for their health. As if there aren't enough reasons to quit already, smoking is the one behavior that clearly has a negative effect on the progression of MS. A study from Harvard found "that current and past smokers with MS were more than three times as likely as patients who had never smoked to have more rapid progression of their disease." Certain medications such as Chantix or Zyban are available to smokers who want to stop. Excessive drinking also is linked to a shorter life expectancy. Women should not drink more one drink per day and men should not drink more than two drinks per day.

There is some evidence from studies of children with MS that physical health, diet, and sleep may lead to a milder MS course. However, it is also possible that children with relatively mild disease were better able to participate in physical activities and monitor their diet. However, this provides more reason for MS patients to pay attention to these factors.

67. Should I Change My Diet?

One of the most frustrating features of MS is that people feel they have little to no control over it. It develops for no apparent reason, and relapses tend to occur at random, unpredictable intervals. It is natural for patients to do anything they can to give themselves a sense of control over their illness. One of the most common and understandable ways that people do this is by changing their diet. It seems obvious that improving one's diet would lead to improvement in every aspect of one's health, including MS. After all, "you are what you eat."

Despite this, there is no clear evidence that diet has a fundamental impact on the course of the disease. As neurologist Dr. Randall T. Schapiro said, "Diets have been used for MS from time immemorial. If they worked, we wouldn't be still talking about them." Additionally, diets are hard to study. There is no money to be made in studying diets, and it is not possible to "blind" someone to what they are eating, as can be done with trials of medications.

Probably the most famous proponent of a dietary treatment for MS was Dr. Roy Swank. He proposed a dietary regimen low in saturated fat as the core feature of his suggested plan, The Swank diet recommends the following:

- No red meat for 1 year—and only minimal amounts afterward.
- Saturated fat should be less than 15 grams per day; unsaturated fats should be 20 to 50 grams per day. Processed food should not contain saturated fat.
- Dairy products should contain 1% or less fat.
- Omega-3 in the form of fish oils are suggested as well as vitamin and mineral supplements.

Dr. Swank published his results in 1990 in the medical journal *The Lancet*, one of the most prestigious medical journals. This article reported on 144 patients who ate a low-fat diet for 34 years. Dr. Swank found that "For each of three categories of neurological disability (minimum, moderate, severe), patients who adhered to the prescribed diet (less than or equal to 20 g fat/day) showed significantly less deterioration and much lower death rates than did those who consumed more fat than prescribed (greater than 20 g fat/day)."

So what does one make of these results? They sure sound impressive. Should every patient with MS radically change their diet as a result of this study? Most neurologists would say "no," as the study is far from conclusive.

First of all, it was not a controlled trial. This means that subjects were not randomly assigned to try his diet or not. Instead, they chose whether or not to participate. This means that only people with significant will-power were able to adhere to his diet, and it is possible that other aspects of this will-power led them to have improved outcomes. Such subjects may have been less likely to smoke, for example, compared to subjects who could not conform to the diet, and smoking is a known risk-factor for worsening disease. They may have been more likely to exercise as well.

Another possibility is that patients whose MS worsened simply gave up on the diet, feeling that it was not working. Thus, patients who had naturally more benign MS may have had an easier time adhering to the diet, rather than the diet causing them to have benign MS. Additionally, no one in the study was blinded. This means that the subjects and evaluators knew what sort of diet they were eating. Thus, subjects may have been motivated, both consciously and unconsciously, to minimize their MS symptoms. Similarly, the examiners grading the subjects may have suffered from similar motivations in evaluating the disability of the subjects. Also, compliance with the diet was based on subjects' reports, and there is no way to verify the accuracy of their reports.

There have been several subsequent studies that investigated the relationship between diet and MS. These studies were recently summarized by the Cochrane Library, a database that reviews and summarizes the results of medical studies to draw overall conclusions about a variety of different topics. This database tends to only summarize trials that are large and without significant methodological flaws. It noted that most studies of diet and MS were of such poor quality that in many cases no meaningful conclusions could be drawn from them. From the studies they did examine, the Cochrane Library concluded that:

> Polyunsaturated fatty (PUFAs) seem to have no major effect on the main clinical outcome in MS (disease progression), but they may tend to reduce the frequency of relapses over two years. However, the data that are available are insufficient to assess a real benefit or harm from PUFA supplementation because of their uncertain quality.

Smaller studies in 2016 and 2017 unsuccessfully attempted to demonstrate the effectiveness of low-fat plant-based and other "healthy diets" in reducing relapses and disability, though one small study found that patients who adhered to such a diet had less fatigue. Terry Wahls, a doctor with a large media presence and online store, claims to have *reversed* her MS with a "paleo" diet and supplements. However, despite dramatic "before and after" pictures, she has no scientific evidence to support her claims that this works for other patients. Clearly more research is needed, and I hope that some of these diets will ultimately yield real benefits for MS patients. But until the science is there to back up treatment claims, I caution patients to use common sense and temper expectations about anecdotal results that sound too good to be true.

So, what is a patient with MS to do regarding diet? First, the vast majority of patients with MS have relatively healthy diets to begin with. Newly diagnosed patients are usually young, fit, healthy people who exercise and don't eat fast food all the time. Conversely, outside of the pediatric age-group, people who eat junk food all the time and don't exercise do not have a higher risk of MS.

This does not mean eating a healthy diet is unimportant. We should all eat proper portions, plenty of fruits and vegetables, and we should all lay off the junk food, though I know how hard this can be! People who eat unhealthy diets and don't exercise are at risk for multiple obesity-related diseases. Even if a healthy diet does not directly impact MS, it will help patients with their waistline and overall health. After all, the most common causes of death in MS are heart disease and cancer, the exact same causes as people without MS. Both of these (especially heart disease) can be modified with a healthy diet.

As such, the dietary advice for people with MS is no different than for people without MS. For this reason, I suggest the Mediterranean diet. It has been shown to reduce the risk of heart disease, diabetes, and even cancer. Key components of the Mediterranean diet are:

- Eat plant-based foods, such as fruits, vegetables, whole grains, legumes, and nuts
- Use olive and canola oil
- Use herbs and spices instead of salt
- Eat fish and poultry at least twice a week while eating red meat only a few times per month
- Drinking red wine in moderation is allowed
- Some exercise every day is a must

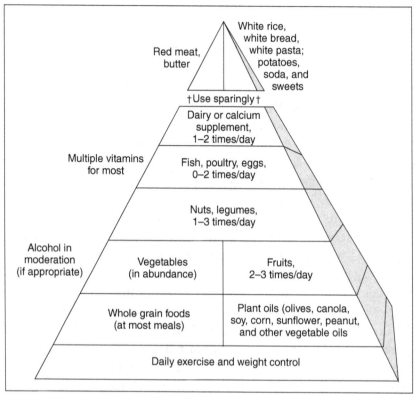

The Mediterranean diet.

As much as possible, I want patients to try to lead the lives they led prior to their diagnosis. I don't want them to adopt fad diets. Yet, due to unfounded fears that food could worsen their MS, some patients develop monk-like lifestyles. They feel they are made of glass and will shatter if they don't eat "just right." I strongly discourage this. At the most extreme, some patients even develop a condition called orthorexia. This is an eating disorder where people feel they have to eat the *perfect* diet. They avoid foods that contain gluten, dairy, meat, sugar, GMOs, soy, lectin, and countless other generally harmless ingredients. Some people spend much of their lives consumed by thinking about food, preparing meals, and feeling guilty if they stray from strict dietary requirements. If they suffer a relapse or worsening of their MS they often blame themselves, feeling a terrible burden of undeserved guilt.

In summary, MS patients should enjoy food like anyone else. It is, after all, one of life's great pleasures. The best dietary advice is from the writer Michael Pollan who wrote: "Eat food, not too much, mostly plants."

68.   *Should I Get the Flu Vaccine?*

Yes, you should get the inactivated flu vaccine. There is no evidence that the flu vaccine is dangerous for people with MS, and there is plenty of evidence that the flu itself is very dangerous. Studies have shown that the flu increases the rate of hospitalizations, relapses, and even mortality in patients with MS. Patients should also insist that their relatives and co-workers get the vaccine. There is a theoretical concern that live vaccines might be unsafe. These vaccines include the influenza nasal spray (FluMist), chickenpox, shingles, and the measles/mumps/rubella (MMR) vaccine. However, no danger from these vaccines has been demonstrated. In fact, only the live vaccine against yellow fever has been shown to be unsafe in MS.

Several of the medications used in MS can predispose patients to shingles, which is the painful reactivation of the virus that causes chickenpox (varicella zoster virus). Occasionally, this virus can lead to serious complications such as strokes. So everything should be done to try to prevent shingles. A new, highly effective shingles vaccine was recently approved for people over the age of 50 years.

So, unless patients are on medications that may suppress the immune system (such as Tysabri, Lemtrada, Ocrevus, and Gilenya), I suggest that they get these suggested vaccines. Ideally, patients should receive all necessary vaccines before starting on their MS medication, as some of the medications may reduce the natural response of the immune system to vaccines.

Additionally, the subject of whether vaccines cause MS has been studied extensively. Despite diligent searching, there is no evidence that any vaccine triggers MS.

69.   *Should I Stop Working?*

Many patients with MS are naturally fearful they will be unable to work, pay their bills, and support their families. Almost all newly diagnosed patients should anticipate that their jobs and schooling can continue uninterrupted for years to come. Patients should continue working unless there is a compelling reason to stop. However, the unfortunate reality is that many patients will have their work affected by their MS. There are several options for people as their relationship with work changes over time:

- Family Medical Leave Act (FMLA)
- Reasonable Accommodations
- Short-Term Disability

- Long-Term Disability
- Social Security Disability Insurance/Supplemental Security Income

Let's go into more detail about each one.

FMLA: It is advised to always have up-to-date FMLA forms on file. This will provide job protection for up to 6 weeks of missed time per year, based on federal law. Patients will also be able to keep their benefits during this time. It can be completed to provide time off intermittently, or in a continuous block. Patients should speak to their Human Resources (HR) Department for the necessary paperwork.

REASONABLE ACCOMMODATIONS: The Americans with Disabilities Act (ADA) requires that employers provide reasonable accommodations for employees with qualifying disabilities. This could include more frequent breaks, relocation of desk space, flexibility to work from home, and office equipment that can make sitting, typing, or performing daily tasks easier.

SHORT-TERM DISABILITY: Patients and their neurologists might agree that a limited break from work can help you to focus on recovery and recuperation. Whether patients have these benefits, and how robust they are, depends on each employer. Patients should speak to their HR Department about what benefits they are entitled to and what paperwork is needed to initiate this process. Short-term disability benefits are granted when it can be shown that patients are temporarily unable to do their job.

LONG-TERM DISABILITY: Whether patients have these benefits depends on their employer. If available, long-term disability would become effective when short-term disability benefits end but patients and their neurologists agree they are still unable to work. Patients should speak to their HR Department about what benefits they are entitled to and what paperwork needs to be completed. Long-term disability benefits are generally granted when it can be proven that patients are unable to do their job.

SOCIAL SECURITY DISABILITY INSURANCE (SSDI)/SUPPLEMENTAL SECURITY INCOME (SSI): Patients and their neurologists might agree that no work at all is possible. As soon as that is decided, an application to SSDI or SSI should be initiated. To qualify as a disabled person for either program, the Social Security Administration (SSA) must agree that the patient is permanently unable to work any job.

- ***SSDI:*** Patients may qualify for SSDI benefits if they have worked long enough to have accumulated a sufficient number of work credits. After receiving SSDI benefits for about 2 years, patients will be eligible for Medicare.

- ***SSI:*** SSI is a needs-based program. If patients meet the SSAs income and asset limits and do not qualify for SSDI, SSI may be the right program for them. If patients are eligible for SSI based on their income and assets, they should also qualify for Medicaid in their state.

No one can say exactly when it is appropriate for someone with MS to stop working. Some patients should clearly go on disability as they are disabled to such an extent that no work is possible. However, many patients continue to go to work, even if they are wheelchair-bound. The ability to work with a disability obviously varies greatly from jobto job.

The decision to stop working should not be made lightly. While disability sounds attractive to many people, work often provides a schedule, a sense of purpose, and valuable social interactions. Many patients who stop working say they've become bored, isolated, and that every day of the week is the same to them. Once people have been out of the work force for some time, it is very difficult to return.

Lastly, patients should disclose their diagnosis at work only when it is helpful to them. No one should disclose due to pressure or guilt. That being said, patients will often need to disclose their diagnosis to their HR Department if they need accommodations or time off.

7

PREGNANCY AND MS

70. How Does Pregnancy Affect the Course of MS?

Unfortunately, MS often strikes women in the prime of their lives when they are thinking of starting a family. In the past women with MS were advised not to get pregnant, as it was thought that pregnancy would worsen their disease. Fortunately, this is not the case. In fact, pregnant women usually have fewer relapses, especially during the second and third trimesters. Indeed, the number of relapses during pregnancy is fewer than the number of relapses expected when taking disease-modifying medications. In contrast, the first months after delivery are a time of increased disease activity. Overall, pregnancy does not have a long-term impact on disability.

While MS itself does not pose a risk to babies, as women gain more weight, some may become less steady while walking. Urinary tract infections are also common, and these must be treated promptly to prevent risk to both the mother and her baby. Bowel problems may also be aggravated in women who experienced them prior to pregnancy. It is also likely that women with MS will experience more fatigue during pregnancy.

Fortunately, the reproductive system is one area that is unscathed by MS. Fertility and fetal development are completely normal in MS. Women with MS do not have a higher risk of having a miscarriage or a still-born child. MS also does not result in an increase in the number of infant deaths or fetal malformations.

In general, I advise women to make a decision to get pregnant independent of their MS. While I realize that this is easier said than done, my goal is to have MS impact their life as little as possible. It would be hard to imagine a greater disruption to a woman's life than deciding not to become a mother because of MS.

71.   What About Fertility Treatments?

Several studies demonstrate that assisted reproduction technology can have a deleterious effect in MS. The medications used in in-vitro fertilization (IVF) therapy may increase relapse risk and increase the number of active, enhancing lesions on the MRI. Still, some women who have trouble conceiving on their own may reasonably decide that the joy of having a baby is worth the increased risk of an MS relapse. There is no "right" answer, and it is up to each woman and her doctors to judge the risks of IVF versus the benefits of conceiving a child.

72.   How Are Relapses Managed During Pregnancy?

Although less likely during pregnancy, relapses can occur and can be a challenge to manage. Their management depends mostly on their severity. Mild relapses may not require treatment, while more severe relapses may be treated with steroids. In general, steroids are safe during the second and third trimester, but they do cross the placenta and can cause transient immunosuppression. Steroids in the first trimester may increase the risk of cleft palate syndrome.

Plasmapheresis, where the patient's blood is filtered to separate the blood cells from other components in the bloodstream, may be a safe and effective option for pregnant patients with a severe relapse. There are case reports of successful treatment of patients with plasmapheresis during pregnancy, and there is evidence from obstetric literature of using plasmapheresis for several blood disorders.

73.   What About Disease-Modifying Therapies During Pregnancy?

None of the disease-modifying medications for MS have ever been studied in a clinical trial in pregnancy, and they never will be. It is unethical to give pregnant women a medication to see what happens to her and her fetus. However, some women do become pregnant while taking these medications. These women are tracked as carefully as possible, allowing us to draw preliminary conclusions about the safety of various medications in pregnancy. The medications are carefully studied in animals, though often at much higher doses than are given to humans. As such, it is difficult to predict from animal data how a medication might affect a human pregnancy.

Copaxone is the only medication that is considered safe in pregnancy, and there is no evidence that there is any danger from the interferons. In contrast, some of the oral medications seem to be potentially harmful.

Most neurologists generally advise women not to be on any MS medication when pregnant, though this is not a universal rule. Pregnancy and childbirth are complicated enough, and if there are problems, no one wants to feel that they were caused by medications.

Because of this, it is important to consider the risks of going off medications while trying to conceive and during a pregnancy. In addition, the period of lactation also needs to be considered. The most common medications for MS are listed with information that is known about their effects on the unborn child.

INJECTABLE MEDICATIONS

- **Interferons:** There are reports of lower mean birth weight, shorter mean birth height, and preterm birth. However, there are no reports of congenital anomalies, developmental abnormalities, or spontaneous abortions. Most women are advised to stop the medication once pregnancy is achieved. The transfer of the medication into breast milk is present in very small amounts.

- **Copaxone:** There are no adverse effects on offspring at up to 36 times the therapeutic human dose. Surveillance studies in humans did not reveal increased risk of adverse fetal or pregnancy outcomes. Patients at high risk of a relapse may be advised to continue therapy while pregnant. The transfer of Copaxone into breast milk is unlikely.

ORAL MEDICATIONS

- **Gilenya:** In the pregnancy registry of Gilenya, there were 28 live births and five cases of abnormal fetal development. These small numbers do not allow us to draw firm conclusions about Gilenya's safety during pregnancy. However, we should obviously err on the side of caution. Effective contraception is advised while on Gilenya and for 2 months after stopping treatment. Evidence of the drug transferring into breast milk comes from experiments in treated rats.

- **Aubagio:** Aubagio is considered category X in pregnancy, meaning that "the risks involved in use of the drug in pregnant women clearly outweigh potential benefits." This is largely based on animal data, however. Aubagio's pregnancy registry includes 26 live births, and thus far, there is no evidence of any harm to the fetus. It is recommended that women undergo accelerated elimination process with cholestyramine and verification of undetectable blood levels prior to attempting to get pregnant while on Aubagio. Without accelerated elimination procedure, Aubagio can stay in the blood anywhere from 8 to 24 months. An effective birth control method is required for women of child-bearing age while on Aubagio.

- **Tecfidera:** The Tecfidera pregnancy registry included 26 live births. Thus far, there is no indication that the medication is harmful to pregnancies in any way.

INFUSIONS

- **Tysabri:** Observational exposure registration study reported miscarriages rate consistent with baseline rate in the United States. The Tysabri pregnancy registry involved 376 women and 316 live births. Although the overall rate of birth defects was slightly higher than expected, the defects did not demonstrate any obvious drug-related pattern. High-risk mothers have been effectively treated with Tysabri throughout their entire pregnancy. Tysabri is secreted in breast milk and should be avoided while breastfeeding.

- **Lemtrada:** Animal studies demonstrate embryo lethality in mice, lowered offspring lymphocyte counts, reduced number of normal sperm, and increased proportion of abnormal sperm without an effect on fertility. A pre-pregnancy wash out of 4 months before attempting pregnancy is recommended.

- **Ocrevus/Rituxan:** Rituxan is the medication that has been used the longest and has the most information from its global registry, which shows that most pregnancies resulted in uncomplicated, live births. In the pregnancy registry for Rituxan, there were 90 live births. Neither the preterm delivery rate nor the risk of congenital malformations was elevated. First trimester loss occurred in 21%, which is higher than the general population rate of 10% to 15% but consistent with reports of women with autoimmune disease and malignancies. The current recommendation is for a 12 month wash out, although successful, healthy pregnancies have been noted within 3 to 6 months of use. Another study of 102 pregnancies on Rituxan found no major safety concerns within 6 months of pregnancy.

74.   What About Symptomatic Therapies in Pregnancy?

Many of the symptomatic therapies used in MS are not considered safe during pregnancy and the risk during lactation is unknown. Ditropan, which is used for bladder dysfunction, is the only medication that is pregnancy category B, meaning it is safe in animal studies. Women should discuss the use of these medications with their obstetrician and neurologist to determine if the benefits of each medication outweigh the risks.

75.   What About MRIs in Pregnancy?

The contrast agent used in MRIs, gadolinium, should be avoided during pregnancy since it has been shown to be harmful in animals at repeated doses. MRIs without contrast are considered safe. Breast milk should be discarded for 24-hours after receiving gadolinium.

76.   What About Labor and Delivery?

Delivery is generally no more complicated in women with MS than for women without MS. Some women have been known to have trouble recognizing that they are experiencing contractions. This is caused by nerve function reduction where there is a lack of sensation below certain lesions in the body. Fatigue may be higher for pregnant women with MS and sometimes this may mean an increased chance of assisted delivery.

Epidurals (when drugs are injected into the epidural space very close to the spinal cord) and spinal anesthesia (when a local anesthetic is injected into the cerebrospinal fluid) are safe and do not increase the chances of relapse or level of disability after the baby is born. General anesthesia is also safe, and this may be an option for women requiring a caesarean delivery.

77.   What About the Postnatal Period?

Although pregnancy is usually a time where relapses are decreased, there is a 20% to 40% increased risk of relapse in the first 3 to 6 months after the birth. The period after the baby is born is a stressful time for any new parent, and increased relapses can make is harder to bond with and nurse a new baby. If a woman has had a lot of relapses in the year before pregnancy or during pregnancy, or a woman was fairly disabled when she became pregnant, she is at an increased risk of relapse when the baby is young.

Relapses are *not* influenced by breastfeeding, having an epidural analgesia, age, or whether or not the woman has had previous pregnancies. Relapses tend to be more severe than previously experienced, but are no more likely than usual to lead to permanent disability. After 6 months, relapse rates tend to decline back to the same level as before pregnancy.

78. What About Breastfeeding?

Breastfeeding is safe in MS, and women who decide not to take a medication in order to breastfeed their baby should know that they are likely not putting themselves at risk of their MS worsening. In fact, there is some evidence that women who breastfeed have fewer relapses than those who don't. In one study of 201 women, 38% who did not breastfeed exclusively had a relapse within the first 6 months after giving birth, while only 24% of women who intended to breastfeed exclusively for at least two months had a relapse. There is evidence that women with clinically isolated syndrome (CIS) have a lower risk for developing clinically definite MS if they breastfeed their babies.

If a woman does experience a relapse while breastfeeding, steroids are safe, though women are advised to pump and discard breast milk for 8 hours after the infusion.

A decision must be made after the baby is born whether women should restart their disease-modifying medication. Studies show that mothers with more active MS generally choose not to breastfeed and return to their usual medicines. This also means that feeding the baby during the night can be shared between both parents. The preference for breast or bottle-feeding is a personal one and the arguments for and against breastfeeding need to be considered carefully. Your neurologist can be helpful in talking about the relative advantages and disadvantages in your own situation.

The Pros and Cons of Breastfeeding in MS

CONS of Breastfeeding	PROS of Breastfeeding
No protection of medicine at a time when relapse is more likely	Many women find emotional connection and meaning in nursing and breastfeeding their baby
Fatigue is worse among women with MS	Does not exacerbate relapses
Fatigue can reduce milk production	You will not pass MS onto your baby via breastfeeding
It may be difficult to support your baby if you experience numbness or weakness in your hands or arms	

GLOSSARY

Axon: The part of a neuron that extends from the cell body, allowing neurons to communicate with each other. Axons are coated with myelin, which is the main site of injury in MS.

Central Nervous System (CNS): The brain and the spinal cord comprise the CNS. The CNS is affected in MS, while the peripheral nerves in the limbs are spared.

Clinically Isolated Syndrome (CIS): Patients who have had just one relapse are said to have CIS. If certain findings are present on either the MRI or in the cerebrospinal fluid, patients with one clinical event can be diagnosed with MS.

Expanded Disability Status Scale (EDSS): The EDSS is the 10-point rating scale used to measure disability in MS.

Lhermitte's Sign: An electrical shock-like sensation that occurs with neck flexion. It is due to pathology of the cervical spinal cord.

Magnetic Resonance Image (MRI): An MRI is a magnet that allows neurologists to visualize both old and new lesions in MS.

Myelin: Myelin is a protective coating of axons composed of fats and lipids. Myelin is made by cells called oligodendrocytes. Myelin allows electrical impulses to move much faster along axons, allowing for rapid communication between cells.

No Evidence of Disease Activity (NEDA): NEDA occurs in patients who have no relapses, no disability progression, and no new MRI lesions.

Oligoclonal Bands: Oligoclonal bands are a marker of inflammation in the spinal fluid found in about 90% of patients with MS. They are not specific for MS and can be found in other diseases.

Optic Neuritis: Inflammation of the optic nerve characterized by partial loss of vision and pain with eye movement.

Primary Progressive MS (PPMS): PPMS is characterized by steadily worsening neurological function or disability from the onset of symptoms. To diagnosis PPMS, there must be 1 year of disease progression.

Progressive Multifocal Leukoencephalopathy (PML): PML is a viral infection of the brain caused by the JC virus, a very common and usually harmless virus. It can be a devastating, even fatal infection. Patients on Tysabri are most vulnerable.

Pseudorelapse: A pseudorelapse occurs when old symptoms worsen in the setting of an infection, fever, or stress.

Relapse: A relapse refers to the rapid onset of neurological symptoms seen in MS. Relapses must last more than 24 hours. They are also called flares, attacks, or exacerbations.

Relapsing-Remitting MS (RRMS): RRMS is the most common type of MS, occurring in over 90% of patients. It refers to the tendency of an MS symptom to start abruptly (a relapse) and then to gradually abate (a remission).

Secondary Progressive MS (SPMS): SPMS follows relapsing-remitting MS after about 15 to 20 years. In SPMS, there is a slow but steady increase in the level of disability. Relapses either disappear completely or occur very rarely.

Uthoff's Phenomenon: The tendency of heat to temporarily worsen MS symptoms.

INDEX

CPSIA information can be obtained
at www.ICGtesting.com
Printed in the USA
LVHW021623070619
620541LV00012B/259/P

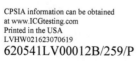